YOU WERE MADE FOR A GARDEN

C·R·E·A·T·I·O·N Health

LIFE GUIDE #3

For Individual Study and Small Group Use

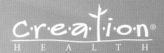

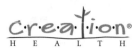

CREATION Health Life Guide #3
Copyright © MMXII by Florida Hospital
Published by Florida Hospital Publishing
900 Winderley Place, Suite 1600
Maitland, Florida 32751

To Extend *the* Health *and* Healing Ministry *of* Christ

Publisher and Editor-in-Chief:	Todd Chobotar
Managing Editor:	David Biebel, DMin
Production:	Lillian Boyd
Promotion:	Laurel Prizigley
Copy Editor:	Mollie Braga
Photographer:	Timothy Brown
Design:	Carter Design, Inc.
Peer Reviewers:	Amaryllis Sanchez-Wohlever, MD; Robert Hayes
	Rev. Robert Schmalzle, MDiv, MSW; Eli Kim, MD
	Andy McDonald, DMin; Gerald Wasmer, MDiv
	Paul Campoli, MDiv; Barbara Olsen, MACL
	Rick Szilagyi, DMin; Andre VanHeerden
	Tim Goff, MDiv; Sabine Vatel, DMin

For volume discounts please contact special sales at:
HealthProducts@FLHosp.org | 407-303-1929

Printed in the United States of America.
PR 14 13 12 11 10 9 8 7 6 5 4 3 2 1
ISBN: 978-0-9839881-7-5

For more life-changing resources visit:
FloridaHospitalPublishing.com
Healthy100Churches.org
CREATIONHealth.com
Healthy100.org

CONTENTS

DOWNLOAD YOUR FREE LEADER RESOURCE

Are you a small group leader? We've created a special resource to help you lead an effective CREATION Health discussion group. Download at: **CREATIONHealth.com/LeaderResources**

WELCOME TO CREATION HEALTH

Congratulations on your choice to use this resource to improve your life! Whether you are new to the concept of CREATION Health or are a seasoned expert, this book was created for you. CREATION Health is a faith-based health and wellness program based on the Bible's Creation story. This book is part of a Life Guide series seeking to help you apply eight elegantly simple principles for living life to the full.

The letters of the CREATION acronym stand for:

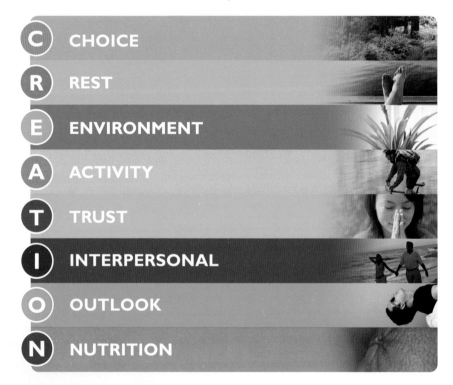

C CHOICE

R REST

E ENVIRONMENT

A ACTIVITY

T TRUST

I INTERPERSONAL

O OUTLOOK

N NUTRITION

In John 10:10 Jesus said, "I have come that they may have life, and have it to the full" (NIV). The Greek word used for life is "zoe," which means the absolute fullness of life…genuine life…a life that is active, satisfying, and filled with joy.

That is why CREATION Health takes a life-transforming approach to total person wellness – mentally, physically, spiritually, and socially – with the eight universal principles of health. Where did these principles come from?

The book of Genesis describes how God created the earth and made a special garden called Eden as a home for his first two children, Adam and Eve. One of the first and finest gifts given to them was abundant health. By examining the Creation story we can learn much about feeling fit and living long, fulfilling lives today.

As you begin this journey toward an improved lifestyle, remember that full health is more than the absence of disease and its symptoms. It's a realization that God desires each of his children – people like you and me whom he loves and cares about – to have the best that this life can offer. It is trusting that your Creator has a plan for your life.

Is there any good parent who doesn't want the best for their child? No. So it makes sense that God would want his best for us. Naturally, human freedom of choice sometimes makes life messy, so not everything can or will be perfect as it once was. But that doesn't mean we shouldn't take a good look at the earliest records of humans found in the Bible to see if there is something special that can be gleaned.

This book – and the other seven in the Life Guide series – takes a deep dive into CREATION Health and translates the fundamental concepts into easy-to-follow steps. These guides include many questions designed to help you or your small group plumb the depths of every principle and learn strategies for integrating the things you learn into everyday life. As a result, you will discover that embracing the CREATION Health prescription can help restore health, happiness, balance, and joy to life.

The CREATION Health Lifestyle has a long, proven history of wellness and longevity – worldwide! People just like you are making a few simple changes in their lives and living longer, fuller lives. They are getting healthy, staying healthy, and are able to do the things they love, well into their later years. Now is the time to join them by transforming your habits into a healthy lifestyle.

If you would like to learn more about the many resources available, visit **CREATIONHealth.com**. If you would like to learn more about how to live to a Healthy 100, visit **Healthy100.org** or visit **Healthy100Churches.org**.

Welcome to CREATION Health,

Todd Chobotar
Publisher and Editor-in-Chief

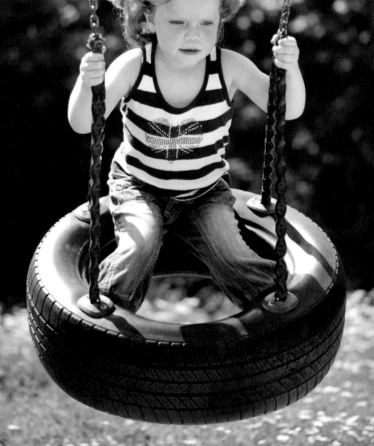

THE ENVIRONMENT WITHIN

LESSON ONE

WARM UP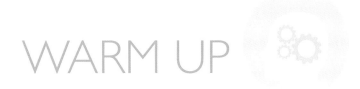

Choose one or both questions to discuss (if in group setting) or write out your answers on a separate sheet (for individual use, in which case question 1 will not apply):

1. **Stand and line up alphabetically by first name.[1] Next, line up alphabetically according to the name of the city/town where you grew up.**

....
....
....
....
....
....

2. **What drew you to this study?[2]**

....
....
....
....
....
....

> *"Whether it's the majestic backdrop of the Rocky Mountains, beach sand squishing between your toes, or the heady fragrance of candles around your bathtub, environment sets the stage for healing of the human soul."*
>
> **MONICA REED, MD**

DISCOVERY

This series of lessons is about the third letter in the CREATION health acronym, E, which stands for the Environment we function in every day, at home, work, and elsewhere. The definition as it is used here is not about climate. It includes everything in our immediate surroundings, the context within which we regularly maneuver. These lessons will take you on an exciting journey of discovery and growth as we learn together how to take a more proactive role in creating a life-giving atmosphere in which to function.

This opening lesson explores how to make our outer environment much more uplifting by focusing first of all on changes we can make to the environment *within* – changes to our own attitude and perspective.

Our world is crammed with both natural and man-made items that have the potential to be elevating if we adopt the proper point of view. Perhaps you have heard the proverbial story of the man who was brought to the Grand Canyon by friends. He stood at the rim, gazed out over the magnificent view, and commented detachedly, "So what's the big deal? It's just a big hole in the ground."

It is the way we see our environment as well as the environment itself that determines its impact. We'll examine three key potential adjustments to our viewpoint and perception – (1) *wonder and curiosity,* (2) *thankfulness*, and (3) *purpose*.

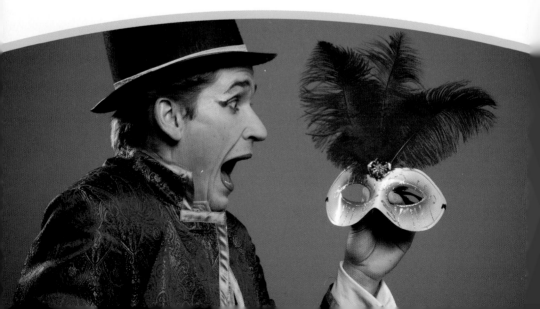

WONDER AND CURIOSITY

To this day, my sister is not sure how she survived having me as an older brother. Her most vivid memory is the time I launched my international career as a seven-year-old magician and convinced her to become my assistant. I was motivated by the magic acts I had seen. They filled me with wonder and a strong desire to know how those mesmerizing tricks were actually done.

For our brother/sister act, I knew we needed something beyond the usual disappearing penny and mystical Chinese ball from the local toy store. To captivate audiences, we needed a grand trick, a real spellbinder.

I chose sword piercing. For swords, I used tapered uprights from an old picket fence. Next I cut matching holes, top and bottom, in an old trunk for the eight swords to pass through. To make the trick work, my sister Sue had to get into the trunk, lay sideways on the floor, and contort herself around the holes to avoid getting jabbed.

It took weeks of practice, but the ultimate effect was quite stunning. For our one and only performance, she entered the "Trunk of Death" waving confidently to the handful of three- and four-year-olds we were able to round up to watch. I closed the trunk lid, uttering the ominous words, "We can only hope that she survives!" I then took each sword, one by one, and, with great flourish, thrust it into the top of the trunk and out the bottom. The gasps from the audience were extremely gratifying.

A measure of that early interest in magic has survived into my married years. In fact, it has evolved into a family tradition. Every Christmas my daughter and I exchange gifts that are reminiscent of our childhood years. I give her a small Lego set and she gives me a simple magic trick. All else on that marvelous holiday would lose some of its luster if that mutual trade didn't take place. Her little gift serves as an annual reminder to never let myself abandon the wonder and curiosity that were such a delightful and essential part of my early years.

> *Our minds and hearts need to periodically flee the shackles of simply surviving.*

When we grow up, the tendency is for the press of daily tasks to absorb all of our attention. We focus entirely on accomplishing, doing, and making ends meet. We get completely caught up in the "what" of life and lose our hold on the invigorating pursuit of "how" and "why." We succumb to the erroneous belief that we don't have time to recapture something from such a distant, less nerve-wracking time.

Such thinking tips the scales much too far on the side of utter practicality. Our minds and hearts need to periodically flee the shackles of simply surviving. We need to be lifted above what is purely mundane. Our thoughts shrivel when they are not allowed time to look more deeply and ponder more pensively. Our mental and emotional health depend on the ability to look beyond what is right before us. Such time is not an indulgence but a necessity. It is by cultivating the inner qualities of wonder and curiosity that we transform our multi-faceted environment into a source of personal enjoyment and edification.

> *We get completely caught up in the "what" of life and lose our hold on the invigorating pursuit of "how" and "why."*

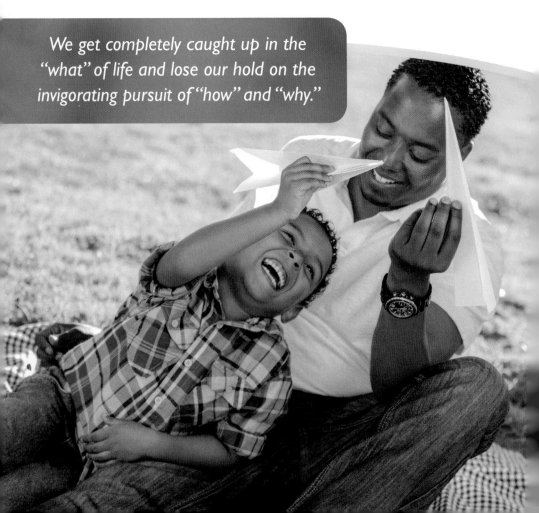

Consider with awe and fascination the everyday items on the list below:

- The intricacies of the African Violet sitting on your side table.

- The incredible infrastructure it takes to allow you to talk to someone in France on your cell phone.

- The immense power of the lightning-filled thunderstorm that boomed and crackled over your house late yesterday afternoon.

- The combination of chemical elements that enable a candle to burn so pleasantly on a dreary Friday evening.

- The Monarch butterfly that somehow migrated hundreds of miles to pause for one delightful moment on your kitchen windowsill.

- The night sky dotted with thousands of stars that are an astounding number of miles away.

- The wonder of a book filled with markings we call letters that carry an author's thoughts across time and space to alter people's thinking.

- The amazing ability of your fingers to apply just the right amount of pressure to pick up a glass of cranberry juice during breakfast.

- The visual cortex in the brain that turns electrical signals from your eyes into complex, multi-colored, 3D images.

- The miracle of spring with life happily bursting out on every hand.

- The micro-chip the size of a speck that connects you to everything.

You might pause for a moment and make up your own list of amazing things in your own environment!

Our immediate world is so complex and intricate that even the smallest, seemingly insignificant component can uplift and move us if we take the time to investigate and understand it. Two of my favorite quotes on wonder are from E. Merrill Root and Jeanette Winterson, respectively:

"We need a renaissance of wonder. We need to renew, in our hearts and in our souls, the eternal poetry, the perennial sense that life is miracle and magic."[3]

"They say that every snowflake is different. If that were the world go on? How could we ever get up off our knee we ever recover from the wonder of it?"[4]

THANKFULNESS

In a broad-based survey, people from various parts of the world were asked to rank their sense of happiness and well-being from 1 to 7, with 1 meaning "not at all satisfied with my life" and 7 meaning "completely satisfied." Among multi-millionaires in America who responded, the average happiness score was 5.8. Pretty good, but you'd think it might be a little higher considering their wealth.

Among the other groups that turned in scores of 5.8 were the Inuits of northern Greenland and the Masai of Kenya. The Inuits number about 55,000 and make their living primarily through hunting and fishing. Because most of Greenland is covered with ice, the Inuits have to settle on the coast where the climate is still harsh. Unemployment is high and their diet is very limited consisting mostly of meat and fats due to the very short growing season. A family's primary possessions are a tent, coverings, and a sled.[5] The dung huts of the Masai have no electricity or running water.[6]

The living conditions of the multi-millionaires are vastly better than those of the Inuits or Masai, yet they have the same happiness score! Clearly satisfaction in life does not depend on our possessions. So rather than wishing for more things, we can simply be thankful for what we already have.

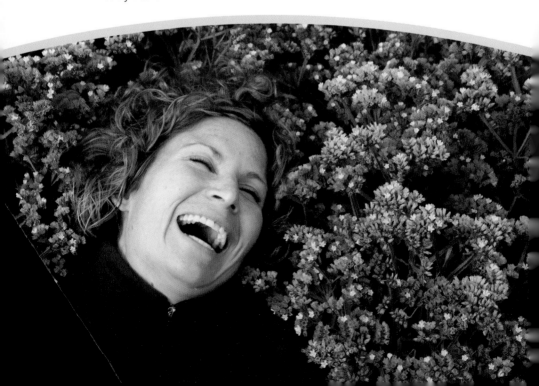

For the following things we can offer sincere thanks:

- Shelter from wind and rain.

- Clothes in our closet, no matter how few or how out of fashion they may be.

- Shampoo that cleanses *and* conditions.

- Clean tap water.

- Warmth from the furnace.

- Intricately designed shells from the beach that grace the knickknack shelf in the hallway.

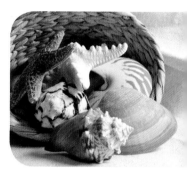

- Birds that sing their little hearts out.

- Nourishing food at our fingertips.

- Our imagination that allows us to explore countless scenarios beyond current reality.

- Muscles and tendons that enable us to bend and move in so many useful ways.

- Our five senses that interact so intimately with our surroundings.

- Children screaming with delight at the antics of a shaggy dog.

- White-crested waves crashing on a wide, sandy shore.

- Complex music that inspires and soothes.

- Family and friends who grace us with love and joy.

- Spiritual insights that offer hope and purpose.

You might pause for a moment and think of some things in your environment you are thankful for.

All of these various aspects of our environment, and many, many more, can evoke within us an ongoing sense of gratitude. Pervasive thankfulness is a powerful emotion that can transport us to a happier, calmer, more fulfilling life.

PURPOSE

One of the most profound verses in Scripture was penned by the apostle Paul, "Therefore, whether you eat or drink, or whatever you do, do all to the glory of God" (1 Cor. 10:31, NKJV). Among other things, Paul is saying that God can be a part of every aspect of our lives, even what we have for breakfast! Doing "all to the glory of God" means doing everything with God-awareness, with a sense of his presence and purposes in mind.

This idea is counter-intuitive to the pervasive concept that the lives of Christians are divided into *sacred* and *secular*. Unbiblical thinking says that we go to our secular job and go about our secular routines at home such as cleaning and paying bills. Then at times we participate in spiritual activities such as Bible study, prayer, and worship. Paul shouts "No!" He says the entire life of a Christian is sacred, not just part of it. It's all included.

So peeling potatoes becomes an act of worship when you do it to strengthen the body God gave you and feed others. When you clean the toilet, it is a sacred task when done to please God by protecting yourself and others from germs. When you sit at your desk at work and process papers, you are participating in one of the "whatever you do" activities Paul talked about that glorifies God. Doing your work with excellence and care becomes just as sacred an activity as singing hymns and prayer.

Jesus turned a carpenter shop into a spiritual place by doing his work with faithfulness and honesty and by loving everyone who entered. He was just as surely honoring God when hammering a wagon wheel together as when he gave the Sermon on the Mount.

In the Old Testament, Joseph turned a prison cell into a sacred place where he glorified God by being faithful and by blessing those around him. He spent two years in a dreadful environment after being falsely accused. He certainly could have become bitter and depressed. But he knew that the daily toil of prison life, with all of its miserable chores, fit within the parameters that God inspired Paul to write about centuries later.

Such an understanding has profound implications for how we relate to our own environment. No aspect of our lives is meaningless. No endeavor is so mundane or routine that it is outside of God's interest and care. Everything in our environment gets uplifted and recast. It becomes part of the complex, stunning tapestry of our lives. There are no common or needless threads. With this awareness, we can now engage our environment with greater interest, satisfaction, and sense of purpose.

Paying attention to the "environment within" by cultivating a sense wonder and curiosity, nurturing a spirit of thankfulness, and seeing purpose in everyday activities forms a great foundation for interacting with the environment around us in meaningful ways.

> *Doing your work with excellence and care becomes just as sacred an activity as singing hymns and prayer.*

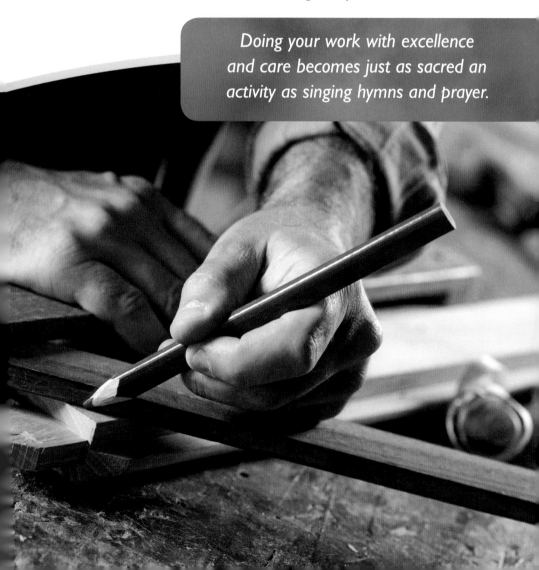

DISCUSSION

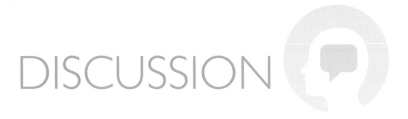

Describe one thing you were especially curious about as a child. What did you learn?

....
....

Was there a time during this last month when you either said or thought "Wow!"? Describe.

....
....

Look at your watch. Can you think of anything amazing about your watch and what it does?

....
....

Share one thing they are thankful for about bread.

....
....

Can we make the choice to be grateful even if we don't feel like it? Is that faking it or not?

....
....

If all of life is sacred for the Christian, how might that impact your attitude throughout the day?

....
....

How can we turn commonplace tasks into acts of worship to God?

....
....

You walk into Jesus' carpenter shop at 11 a.m. on a Wednesday morning. What specifically is he doing? Describe his facial expression and body language the moment he sees you.

....
....

SHARING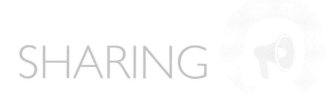

OPPORTUNITY #1

This section is about an opportunity for you to be a blessing to someone outside of your small group and to also deepen the impact of the lesson on your own life. The group is encouraged to discuss at the end of each meeting what aspects of the lesson they might like to share with someone at home, work, or in the community if the opportunity arises. *There is "An Abundant Living Thought" at the end of each lesson as one possibility of something to pass along.*

Start each day asking God to provide opportunities to share and then keep your radar up.

You can be an ambassador and reach people with the good news that abundant living is available to all.

ABUNDANT LIVING THOUGHT

Our thoughts shrivel when they are not allowed time to look more deeply and ponder more pensively.

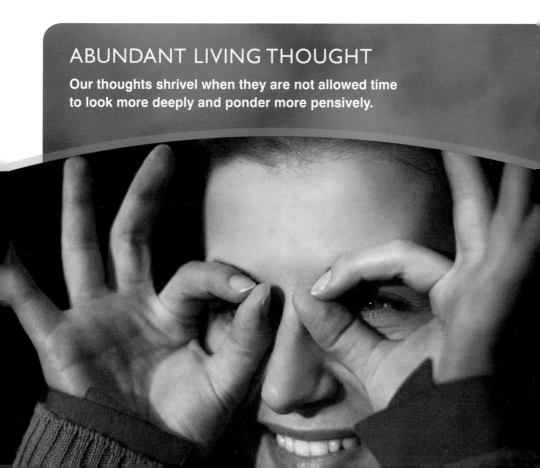

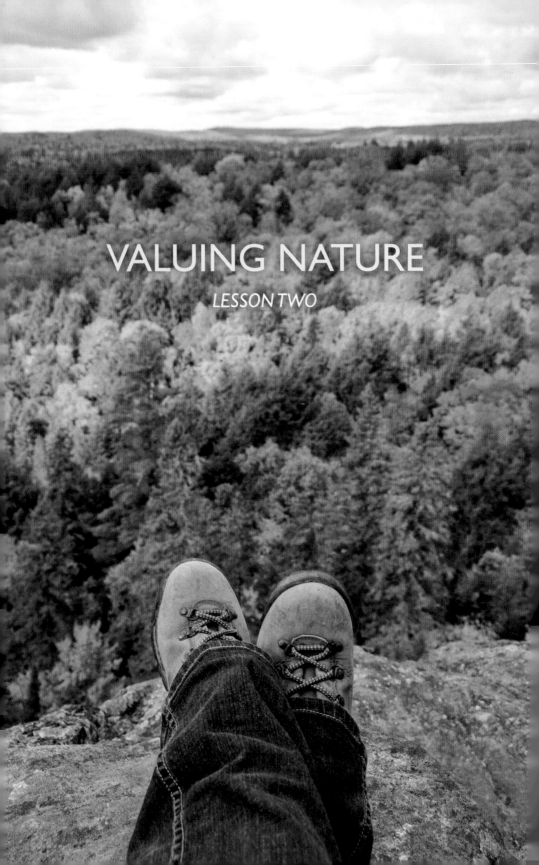

VALUING NATURE

LESSON TWO

WARM UP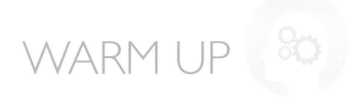

Feedback: In what ways did God open the door last week for you to share some part of the lessons with someone else?

....
....
....
....

Choose one or both questions to discuss (if in group setting) or write out your answers on a separate sheet (for individual use, in which case question 2 will not apply):

1. **Tell about an activity or hobby you enjoyed as a teenager that you don't do now.**

....
....
....
....

2. **Stand in a circle and create a wave like at a sporting event with each person in turn raising both arms overhead. Reverse direction. Create another wave by only laughing in turn. Reverse direction.**

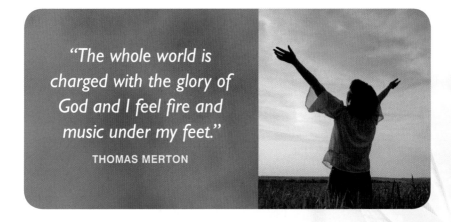

"The whole world is charged with the glory of God and I feel fire and music under my feet."

THOMAS MERTON

DISCOVERY

My mother specialized in baking sweets. In fact, one delicious summer she helped run a bakery in what had been an old, abandoned, red brick railroad station behind our house. All during my childhood, she produced a continuous stream of cakes, cookies, and specialty breads.

The ultimate treat was when my mother would bake a phenomenal blueberry pie for me and three of my closest friends. The agreement was that if we picked the blueberries, she'd make the pie. During the short picking season, we would head out about once a week, baskets in tow. The berries grew in knee-high bushes located in a variety of conducive places. Mouths watering, bellies yearning, we gathered the little blue gems with the eagerness of prospectors frantically scratching for gold.

Those memorable pies were made all the more enjoyable because we kids had a hand in producing them. Each melt-in-your-mouth masterpiece was the direct result of our familiarity with all the blueberry hangouts in the countryside around us.

We knew the territory from having spent summers outside in the fields, seashore, woods, and hills. Even during the school year, nature was our second home.

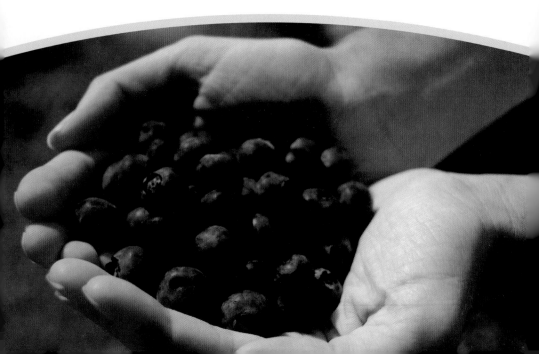

Years later, after starting my own family, our residence was surrounded by woods, about 150 feet back from the road. Deer, moose, and birds of every description blessed our acreage.

Many weekends were spent climbing mountains with our daughter in New Hampshire's Presidential Range. Nothing compares to laboring for two hours up a steepening incline, then breaking out into the open to enjoy the sweeping view from four thousand feet up. No lunch tastes as good as the one eaten on a mountain overlook on a crisp fall day.

We also spent many weekends as a family patrolling the nearby shoreline investigating the intriguing inhabitants of myriad tidal pools. Now in Florida, we only own a postage stamp of land but often escape to the award-winning state parks.

Science has now made it official – experiencing nature is an important pathway to human health and well-being. We now know that personal involvement with the natural world needs to be a key component of everyone's life-giving environment.

Numerous studies demonstrate that becoming engaged with nature can result in a significant reduction of stress, anxiety, blood pressure, and heart rate, as well as elevating ones mood.[7] Researchers at the Centre for Environment and Society at the University of Essex studied more than 1,850 individuals who got their exercise in natural environments. The researchers called it "green exercise."[8] The results revealed improvements in self-esteem along with reduced feelings of anger and depression.[9] Studies done at the University of Rochester, New York, indicate that exposure to natural settings frequently leads people to nurture closer relationships with others, to value community, and to be more generous.[10]

Healthcare institutions are also catching on to the benefits of bringing patients into contact with nature. At a two-hundred-bed hospital in suburban Pennsylvania, some patients had rooms on the surgical floors that looked out on a stand of deciduous trees while others faced a brown brick wall. Researchers discovered that patients with the tree view had shorter stays by almost one full day, fewer requests for pain medication, and fewer negative comments to nurses. This finding has been replicated in other settings.[11]

Children are especially benefitted by being given the opportunity to learn and play in nature. In 2006, Danish researchers found that kindergartens connected with the outdoors experienced a marked increase in creativity among the children.[12] Another study of over a hundred public high schools in Michigan discovered that students from classrooms and lunchrooms that had large windows with views of natural settings had higher test scores.[13]

When at-risk students were enrolled in weeklong outdoor education programs, they exhibited enhanced cooperation and conflict management skills, improved classroom behavior and problem solving, plus greater motivation to learn.[14] Another survey discovered that children in grades three to five with more nature near their homes suffered from less behavioral disorders, anxiety, and depression.[15] Involvement with nature even has a positive impact on childhood obesity.[16]

The problem is that our society is increasingly becoming disconnected from nature. Kids between ages eight to eighteen spend an average of 6.5 hours a day staring at electronic screens. The number of children involved with hiking, walking, and fishing dropped 50 percent from 1997 to 2003. Eighty percent of young ones under age two and more than sixty percent of those who are ages two to five lack daily outdoor play.[17]

In 2008 the updated edition of *"Oxford Junior Dictionary"* removed the names for over ninety plants and animals, including vine, violet, clover, dandelion, and sycamore. The lexicographers added, "MP3 players, voicemail, blogs, chat rooms, and BlackBerry."[18] A child once commented, "Why would I go outside and play? There aren't any electrical outlets."

Society has devoted enormous amounts of energy to giving people access to every little smidgeon of information around the world but has taught families almost nothing about how to access the life-giving assets of the natural world. Spending time in nature doesn't even show up on most people's radar and we are the poorer for it. In order to correct that imbalance and experience life at its best, we need to believe that *the more technology we embrace, the more nature we need.*

> *Children are especially benefitted by being given the opportunity to learn and play in nature.*

Wouldn't it be wonderful if kids could safely roam and explore today the same way they did during my childhood? During the summer months, each of us ages five and up would head out the door right after breakfast, yelling back at our smiling parents, "See you for lunch." And off we'd go with a gaggle of friends for another day of investigating, playing, climbing, building, racing, experimenting, and observing the outdoors.

Today that's mostly unheard of due to the fear of despicable adult weirdos who harm young ones. That fear is not without merit. But overdone, it can deprive children of the opportunity to develop vital skills and understandings. Kids live through their senses and nature happily and easily calls out to every one of those senses, not only sight and hearing, but also smell, touch, and taste. It engages our feelings of curiosity and wonder like nothing else can. Rather than letting our fears dictate our priorities, we need to find new, creative ways to keep our kids safe and fill their world with nature's essential bounties.

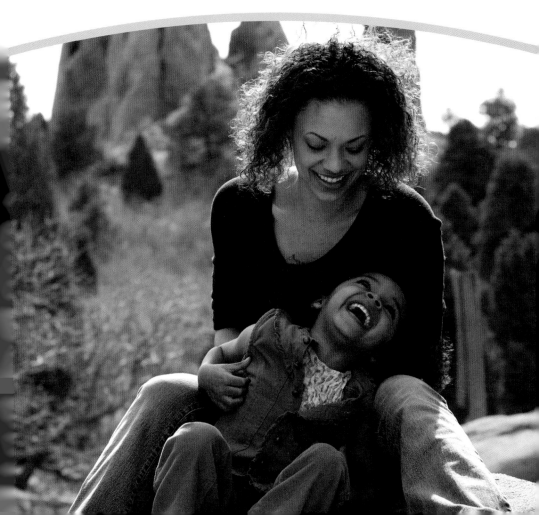

About twenty years ago, my wife, Ann, our daughter Stefanie, and I took a two and half week trip of a lifetime out West from Maine. We camped the whole way except for the two or three times we took refuge in a motel on particularly hot, humid days. We visited the Rockies, Bryce Canyon, the Grand Canyon, and other stunning natural attractions. Stef turned thirteen at the Grand Canyon's North Rim. We had made reservations for dinner at the magnificent lodge. Waiters seated us at floor-to-ceiling windows with exhilarating vistas just as the pink hues of sunset graced the tips of the settling clouds. A sense of wonder characterizes our memories even to this day.

Connecting with nature, however, does not need to involve such grand, large-scale treks. Many marvels of the natural world are as accessible as our own backyards or neighborhoods and can have an especially important impact on children. Richard Louv, founder of the Children & Nature Network, writes, "The dugout in the weeds or leaves beneath a backyard willow, the rivulet of a seasonal creek, even the ditch between a front yard and the road – all of these places are entire universes to a young child. Expeditions to the mountains or national parks often pale, in a child's eyes, in comparison with the mysteries of the ravine at the end of the cul de sac… By expressing interest or even awe at the march of ants across these elfin forests, we send our children a message that will last for decades to come, perhaps even extend generation to generation."[19]

When God created Adam and Eve, he could have housed them in a mansion with ten bedrooms, an elegant living room, expansive family room with marble flooring, high ceilings, and a kitchen fit for a classic French chef. Instead God placed them in a garden called Eden. They shaped the vines, arranged the flowers, spread soft green moss for flooring, and enjoyed stunning, expansive views.

Jesus, the Creator of Eden, left his cozy home in Nazareth at age thirty to live in nature full-time until his death approximately three years later. He occasionally accepted the hospitality of friends, but often seemed to prefer camping out under the stars. Each night, he drifted off to sleep to the sounds of birds and animals he himself had invented. Jesus drew upon those years of outdoor living for his parables about sparrows, lilies, grass, mountains, gardening, and figs, to name a few.

God's preference for nature should tell us something about his value system. The psalmist calls upon nature to praise its Creator and we can join that chorus of appreciation for what he has made: "Let every created thing give praise to the Lord, for he issued his command, and they came into being" (Psalm 148:5, NLT).

> *"People from a planet without flowers would think we must be mad with joy the whole time to have such things about us."*[20]

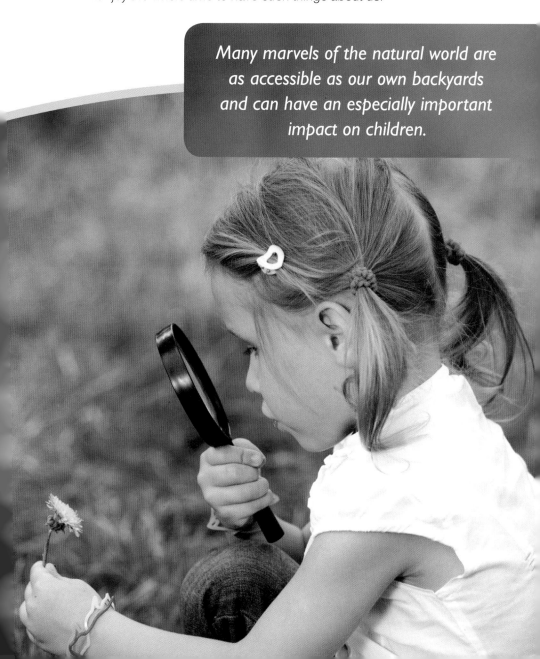

Many marvels of the natural world are as accessible as our own backyards and can have an especially important impact on children.

DISCUSSION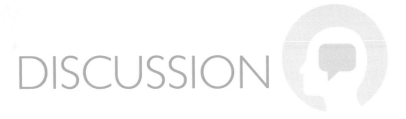

How would you define "nature" using what you've learned from this lesson? Utilizing that definition, give an example of nature close to you.

....

....

As a child, did you spend time in nature? Describe a particular experience that was meaningful for you.

....

....

Which of the benefits of nature described in this lesson caught your interest the most? Why are these benefits valuable to you?

....

....

If you planned a "Nature Day" for yourself and those close to you, what would it include?

....

....

What might help reverse the trend of children spending less and less time in the natural world?

....

....

Would you rather take a tram up a mountain or a boat out to sea? Why?

....

....

If you could become an animal in nature, which one would it be? Why?

....

....

SHARING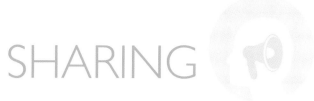

OPPORTUNITY #2

- Pray for God to open the way for you to share something from these lessons to help someone else this week.

- Keep your radar up each day for opportunities.

ABUNDANT LIVING THOUGHT

Experiencing nature is an important pathway to human health and well-being... The more technology we embrace, the more nature we need.

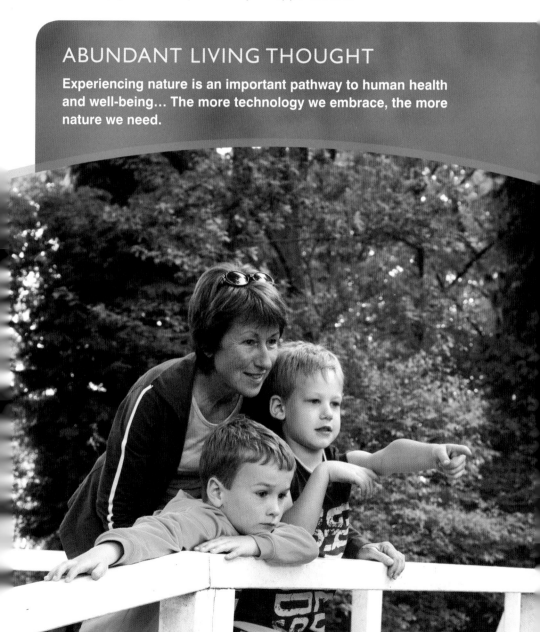

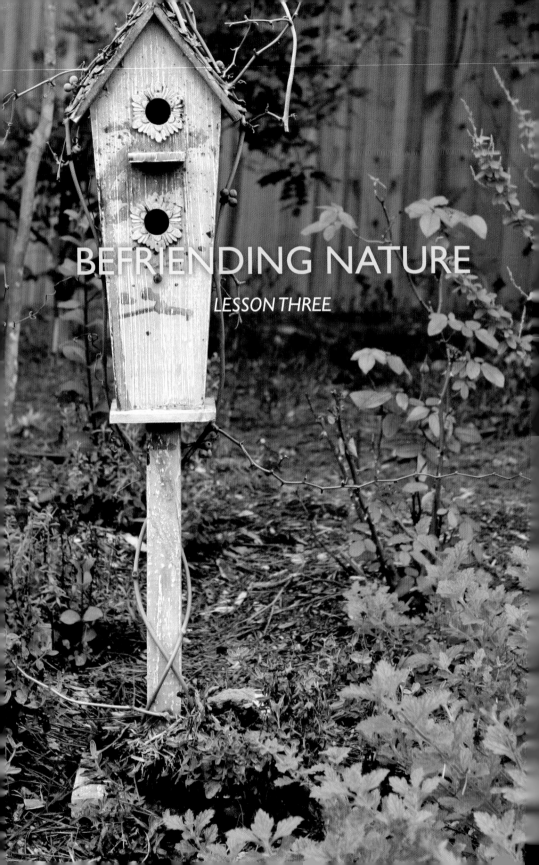

BEFRIENDING NATURE

LESSON THREE

WARM UP

Feedback: In what ways did God open the door last week for you to share some part of the lessons with someone else?

....

....

....

....

Choose one or both questions to discuss (if in group setting)
or write out your answers on a separate sheet (for individual use):

1. **What is the best thing you can imagine happening to you in the next three years?**[21]

    ....

    ....

    ....

2. **Who is the closest friend you had in childhood? Tell about a memorable experience with that person.**[22]

    ....

    ....

    ....

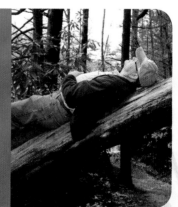

"Immerse yourself in nature. It sooths the soul, clears the mind, and guarantees you a great day!"

DR. DAVID BIEBEL

DISCOVERY

After retiring from his job as a car parts salesman, my father had transformed one third of his small backyard into a lush vegetable garden. Despite a limited area to work in, he patiently coaxed enough lettuce, tomatoes, peppers, radishes, and other produce out of the ground to feed himself, my mom, and the grateful neighborhood. Whenever I visited dad, the garden assumed a prominent place in our conversations, accompanied by a plant by plant tour. Pointing to a particularly energetic piece of greenery, he'd exclaim, "See this one, Bub [he always called me Bub], just last week it was only this tall. Now look at it!" A smile, broad as a cucumber, spread across his rugged, tanned face.

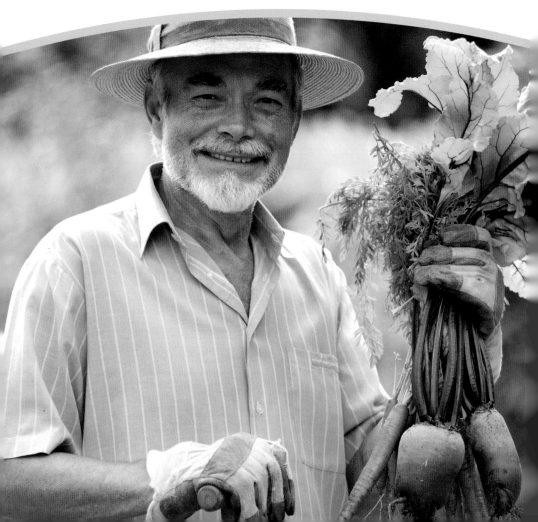

Dad also turned the backyard into a sanctuary for hungry birds. At least half a dozen feeders of various shapes and sizes hung invitingly from the branches of three stately pine trees. He'd never let the supply of food run out any more than he'd let his own refrigerator get empty.

Unfortunately, a gang of brazen squirrels regularly looted every one of the irresistible feeders. Dad groped for an answer. Then, one day, while rummaging around the attic, he found my childhood BB gun, a pump action with BBs still rattling around inside. *Perfect*, he thought.

Early the next morning he pumped the gun to fill it with air and waited behind a bush for the squirrel raiding party. Squirrel #1 unashamedly walked out from behind a tree. Dad's army training kicked in. Blam! The squirrel glanced his way, smiled, then nonchalantly meandered off unharmed. Squirrel #2 appeared. Re-pump. Aim. Blam! That furry critter also sauntered off unscathed. I picture the others lined up on a branch waving and jeering.

Exasperated, my father finally chose to examine the old gun a little closer. He fired it again, and watched as a tiny BB dribbled out the front of the barrel and fell directly at his feet. The tired rifle could no longer create much air pressure. Dad threw the gun down, raised the white flag, and simply filled the feeders more frequently.

I don't endorse my dad's methods. Squirrels are just as valuable as birds. But he would do anything for his beloved feathered friends.

Discovering nature nearby after retirement did wonders for my father. He loved to get his hands in the soil and nurture his splendid crop. It gave him a sense of purpose and great enjoyment. It provided exercise, fresh air, sunlight, and tangible rewards for hard work. He also spent many hours observing the birds and could almost identify them individually. It all renewed and sustained him physically, mentally, and emotionally.

For us today, it's best to become engaged with nature long before retirement. We need to make time to integrate nature's benefits into our lives as early as possible. We should no longer view time spent in nature as leisure and consider it instead as an essential investment in our own happiness and well-being. Making friends with the out-of-doors is a vital part of living life to the fullest.

The following is a series of practical suggestions to help you get more involved with the natural world:

GARDENING

Research has discovered that the simple act of gardening can enhance longevity and benefit overall physical health. Advantages include helping to improve mood, relieve stress, boost low self-esteem, and done regularly, build bone and muscle.[23]

You can be a gardener whether you live on a fifty acre farm or in a city apartment. There are many different types of gardens to choose from:[24]

Hanging Garden – Potted plants hang from various devices that can be attached to walls or ceilings. Perfect for patios and balconies.

Container Garden – Whether indoors or out, plants can thrive in a variety of containers from pots to windowsills.

Mediterranean Garden – These usually have gravel pathways meandering amidst herbs and bright flowers. Nearby walls are often covered with vines.

Monochromatic Garden – Flowers of the same color are grouped together to form swaths of reds, blues, yellows, etc. Choose combinations that fit your fancy.

Oriental Garden – The goal is a feeling of calmness and serenity. This is often achieved by use of water fountains and ponds with open areas of sand or small gravel.

Raised Garden – Raised beds can be made from treated lumber, brick, or stone filled with soil and plants.

Scent Garden – A liberal use of aromatic plants, flowers, and herbs create a wonderfully scented garden.

Tropical Garden – It feels like a piece of the jungle with palms, orchids, vines, and ferns swaying in the breeze.

Whimsical Garden – It is whatever you desire, a bit unruly, somewhat messy, with surprises tucked in along the way.

OTHER NATURE ACTIVITIES

Because connecting with nature is so important for the well-being of both children and adults, we have provided a starter list of potential activities in addition to gardening for those who are looking for creative ways to spend meaningful time outside. Look over the list and choose what you feel might be most appropriate for you and your particular situation. By providing specific examples, we hope to answer the question: *"Aside from gardening or simply walking casually in the woods, what else is there to do?"* The goal is for you to not only learn new facts as you spend time outdoors, but to also experience a deeper sense of joy, serenity, and attachment to the natural world. If you are patient, observant, and receptive, those benefits will come as you learn to view nature as a friend.

A list of outdoor activities for you to choose from:

1. **Collect stones, shells, feathers, pinecones, or leaves.** Learn about them, their similarities and differences. Paint or decorate them. Put them in a prominent place in the house.

2. **Sit in a quiet comfortable place in nature,** be silent, and see how much you can hear. Don't move. Become part of the environment.

3. **Study bird songs and calls.** What birds are they? Try to replicate their sounds. Track how bird sounds differ at various times of the year.

4. **Visit a pond** at night and listen to the frogs.

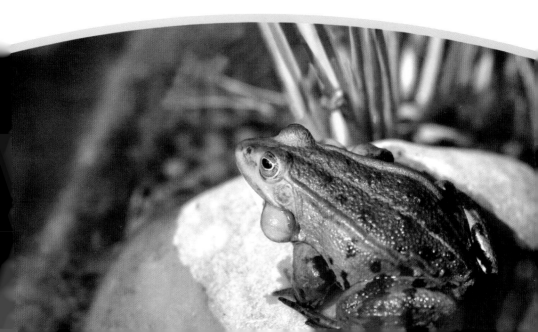

5. **Observe squirrels** in your neighborhood and see if you can discover their favorite routes and hang outs.

6. **Visit the same place in your backyard** once a week and observe what changes. Keep a journal.[25]

7. **Get acquainted with some trees in your area.** What are their characteristics? How do they differ? Measure their growth.[26]

8. **Adopt a piece of the earth.** Find areas that need attention and improve them.[27]

9. **Set aside one hour daily** to play outside in an unstructured way.

10. **Take digital pictures of nature** and make a collection on your computer. Send them to friends. Turn them into wallpaper for your monitor. Frame them for the house.

11. **Camp out in the backyard.** Spend time cloud watching and star gazing.

12. **Feed birds.** Start a birdbath.

13. **Engage older relatives** in your outings. Ask them to share their memories of nature.

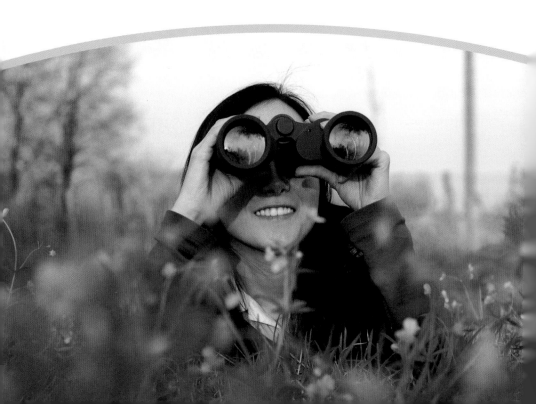

14. **Make a heaping bed of fallen leaves,** pine needles, and natural debris and create a cozy indentation in the middle where you can lie down on your back cocooned in what you have gathered. Nestle in then look up at your surroundings from this new vantage point.[28]

15. **Form pairs and decide which person in each pair will wear a blindfold.** The other person becomes the leader, holding their partner's hand and guiding them on a nature walk. Sight is the sense we depend on most and by taking that out of the equation, our other senses come more alive and engaged. The leader has to watch for logs, slippery places, and low hanging branches. The guide presents the blind partner with interesting objects to feel and smell. After a while, change places.[29]

16. **Have an adult secretly collect ten different items** from the woods and spread them out on a handkerchief. Place another handkerchief over them. Have others, especially children, gather around. Tell everyone that you are going to lift the covering for twenty-five seconds and then place it back. They have ten minutes to find as many of the items themselves as they can. When time is up, dramatically pull each item out from under the handkerchief and see who found them.[30]

17. **Give each person a string about three to five feet long.** Tell them to stretch it over a part of the ground that looks interesting. Then have them get down on their bellies and crawl along the length of the string, examining the ground inch by inch. They must keep their eyes no more than a foot off the ground. Giving each person a magnifying glass greatly enhances the experience. After several minutes, everyone reports their findings by giving others a tour of the area along their string.[31]

18. **Provide each individual with an imaginary deed** to one square mile of land. Ask them to draw a picture representation of their own dream forest on paper with various trees, animals, hills, rivers, caves, etc. Give some suggestions up front to spark their thinking. Discuss each person's plan.[32]

19. **Pin a picture of something in the woods** on the back of a person (animal, rock, tree, stream, etc). Don't show it to them. Have them turn around so everyone else can see it. The person wearing the picture asks questions to discover what they are. Others can only answer yes or no.[33]

20. **Find a scrap board and put it down on bare dirt.** Lift it up in a couple days to see what insects are using it for shelter.[34]

21. **Keep a "Wonder Bowl"** where kids empty their pockets after a nature activity.[35]

22. **Go bird watching or animal tracking.**

23. **Go canoeing or kayaking.**

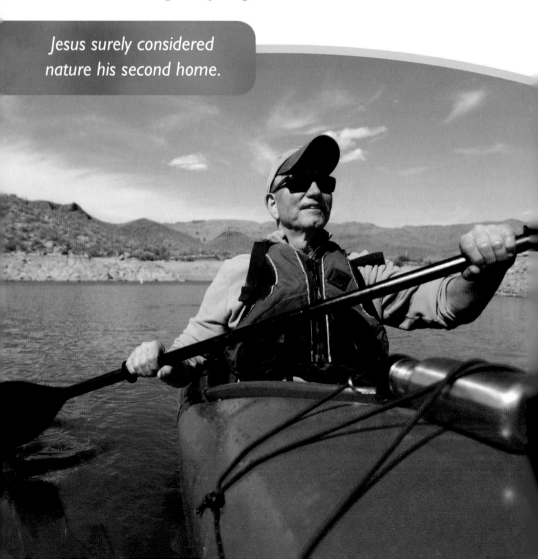

Jesus surely considered nature his second home.

JESUS AND NATURE

During the years prior to his public ministry, Jesus surely considered nature his second home, since his later teachings contained so many illustrations from the flora and fauna of his day.

Jesus' love for the outdoors continued after he left home. I can imagine that he was especially drawn to the gorgeous gardens that many land-owners cultivated in those days. The pleasant sites, calm surroundings, and invigorating aromas would have been a welcome retreat from the press of his daily ministry.

Christ was clearly drawn to the Garden of Gethsemane, located on the slopes of the Mount of Olives near Jerusalem. There were, without doubt, many olive trees there because the word Gethsemane means "olive press." The gospel writer John tells us that Jesus visited there frequently; "Jesus, having prayed this prayer, left with his disciples and crossed over the brook Kidron at a place where there was a garden. He and his disciples entered it. Judas, his betrayer, knew the place *because Jesus and his disciples went there often"* (John 18: 1-2, The Message, emphasis added).

Luke tells us that Christ and the disciples spent every evening of his final Passover Week in Gethsemane, "Each day Jesus was teaching at the temple, and *each evening* he went out to spend the night on the hill called the Mount of Olives" (Luke 21:37, NIV, emphasis added).

Jesus is our example in many areas of life – how to know God, how to treat others, how to be steadfast to principle, to name a few. It is also important to follow Jesus' example regarding his relationship to nature by going there often and viewing time spent there as walking in his sacred steps.

The following is a list of online resources that provide ideas and incentives for getting involved with the outdoors:

- National Wildlife Federation's "Be Out There" initiative at http://www.nwf.org/Get-Outside/Be-Out-There.aspx.

- "Pigeon Watch" at http://www.birds.cornell.edu/pigeonwatch. A helpful book on this topic is *Sharing Nature with Children, 20th Anniversary Edition,* by Joseph Cornell.

- "Nature Rocks: Let's Go Explore," http://www.naturerocks.org/.

DISCUSSION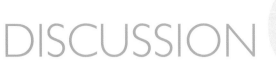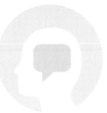

Have you ever had a garden? Please describe it.

....

....

From the list of different types of gardens in the lesson, which one captures your interest the most? Why? How could you start one?

....

....

Do you consider yourself to have a "green thumb" or not? Why?

....

....

Select one of the twenty-three outdoor activities listed in the lesson that you have *already done before.* Describe the experience.

....

....

Pick one of the outdoor activities listed in the lesson that you have *never done before* but would be interested in trying. Explain why you made that choice. How could you get started?

....

....

What kind of seed would you choose to plant? Why?

....

....

Based on the illustrations and parables Jesus used in his teachings, what do you think were some of his favorite parts of nature?

....

....

Which place best captures how you have felt in the last few days? Why?

MOUNTAIN TOP ....

LUSH GARDEN ....

OPEN FIELD ....

VALLEY ....

DITCH ....

....

SHARING

OPPORTUNITY #3:

- Pray for God to open the way for you to share something from these lessons to help someone else this week.

- Keep your radar up each day for opportunities.

ABUNDANT LIVING THOUGHT

We should no longer view time spent in the natural world as leisure and consider it instead as an essential investment in our own happiness and well-being.

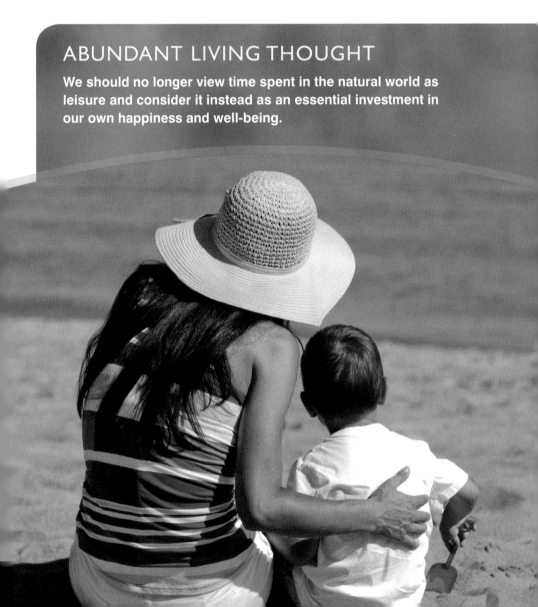

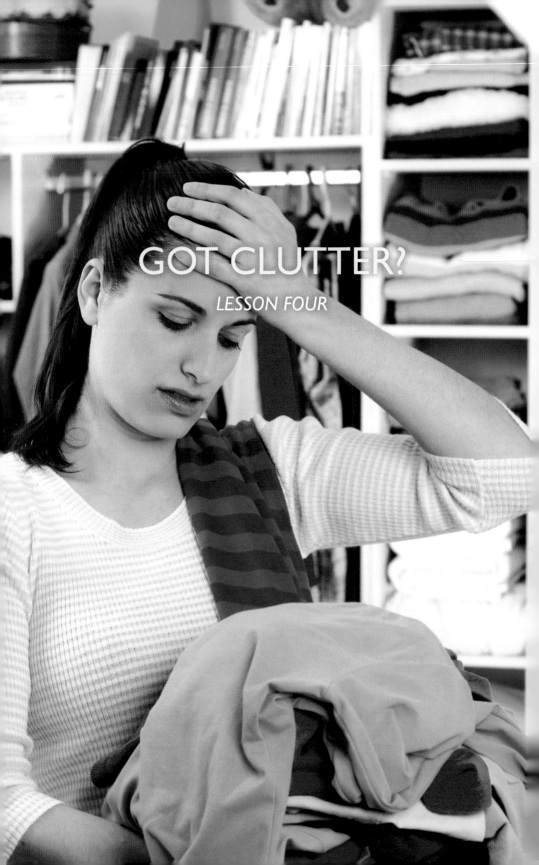

GOT CLUTTER?
LESSON FOUR

WARM UP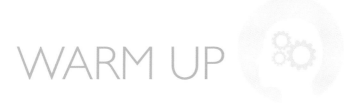

Feedback: In what ways did God open the door last week for you to share some part of the lessons with someone else?

....

....

....

....

Choose one or both questions to discuss (if in group setting) or write out your answers on a separate sheet (for individual use):

1. **Describe a positive change, big or small, you have made in your life in the last two years.**

....

....

....

2. **"What has been one of the most memorable compliments you've received as an adult?"**[36]

....

....

....

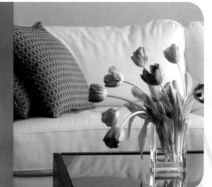

"The ability to simplify means to eliminate the unnecessary so that the necessary may speak."

HANS HOFMANN

DISCOVERY

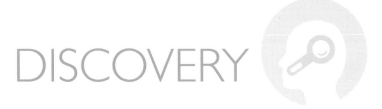

Most people's perception of the word "clutter" has to do with quantity, allowing too many things to encumber a person's living space.

On one end of the spectrum are the extreme hoarders like Eugenia, a sixty-year-old business woman. Her children had no choice but to intervene when they found her sleeping in the yard of her Southern California home. The house was so full of stuff that they could only enter through a window. Trash, pictures, clothes, newspapers, and various other items were piled up about four feet high in room after room. Water leaks meant the bottom layer was rotted and mildewed. It took the children eight weeks and about $20,000 to empty the place out.[37]

On the other end of the clutter spectrum, we might envision people who wrestle with far less accumulation than Eugenia, but nonetheless have tendencies, pieces of the problem. It may be a small pile in a corner of the house or a stack of boxes in the garage.

Actually, clutter, in the broadest sense, is not about quantity at all. A definition that I found particularly helpful is from author Nancy Twigg, *"Anything that has outlived its usefulness in your life… Whether something is clutter depends on what you get out of it."*[38] She goes on to say, "The yardstick for measuring clutter is how much value something gives back in relation to the time, space, and effort it requires."[39]

From that perspective, clutter is not fundamentally about piles, messiness, and disorder. It involves allowing any number of items into our environment that are no longer directly related to our peace, happiness, and sense of well-being. With this definition, even the neatest among us can have clutter issues.

The question is, why do we cling to some items so tenaciously when they have no positive impact on us and have outlived their usefulness? It turns out that there are several internal motivations that drive us in that direction. *Clutter begins inside of us and then expresses itself in outward behaviors.* As one author put it, "Your outer environment is simply a reflection of what's going inside you, inside your mind, in your thoughts and beliefs and consciousness."[40]

This understanding of clutter matters because we are striving to create an environment that will free us rather than constrain us. It matters because our possessions hold clues to what we value and who we are. The more aware we become of the various rationales that people have for creating clutter, the more intelligently we can address the problem.

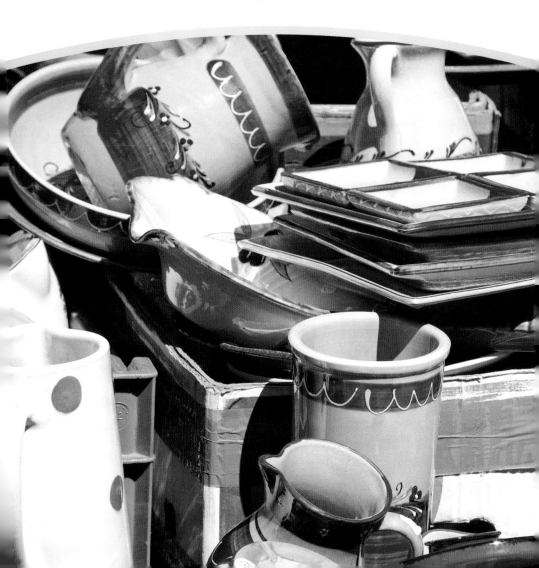

The following list is a brief summary of some of the major reasons people hang onto certain things:[41]

POSITIVE MEMORIES

I have a large box of stuff from my childhood – band hat, the purple and white varsity jacket and white, bulky varsity sweater I got from playing hockey in high school, news clippings about our hockey games, report cards, photos, research papers, correspondence, etc.

Another large box is full of stuff relating to the trip our family took to Cape Breton Island on the east coast of Canada to discover my roots where my grandmother grew up – maps, pieces of glass and pottery we dug up at the old homestead, rocks from the foundation, photos, directions scribbled by my nanny, correspondence with locals, a hand rubbing from a relative's grave, copies of deeds, copies of great grandfather's will, originally written in the flyleaf of his Bible, etc.

I tell myself that these are important memories to hang on to, but the problem is that I never look at any of it. They are simply two more boxes that we dutifully carry from place to place whenever we move. Two more boxes that get stuffed onto a high shelf or piled in a corner of the garage and then sit there like relics from a bygone era.

If they meant so much, why wouldn't I put them on display where they could fulfill an uplifting purpose? The better solution is to take a photo of certain items and then get rid of them all. I could also save one or two items that have the most meaning and toss the rest. This would have the added benefit of releasing me from any lingering notion that my identity is tied up with my possessions.

NEGATIVE MEMORIES

One man kept some trophies he received from his days as a football player in college to remind himself how out of shape he was now in his mid-forties. He hung onto them in an attempt to shame himself into exercising. Research has demonstrated over and over again that negative motivation is rarely effective. Because the trophies do not contribute to a positive frame of mind, they should be tossed.[42]

POSTPONING DECISIONS

My wife and I still laugh about the days when I used to make my annual trek to an office supply store to finally get organized. Once and for all I was going to make the piles of paper that grew like mushrooms in various parts of the den go away. They were going to be forcibly uprooted and relocated to file drawers or the town dump.

I remember wandering the store, searching for the magic solution. A look of fierce determination gathered on my face as I foraged among the aisles. I scanned the options looking for something better than last year's magic solution that had failed to deliver. But no matter what system I tried, the mushrooms always eventually won.

Actually, the real solution couldn't be found in a store. The underlying problem was my anxiety about making decisions regarding what to keep and what to toss. And then having to make decisions about where to file what I kept.

My perfectionism worked against me. Instead of creating a perfectly clean desk, it caused me to put off making any decisions for fear of making the wrong one and never being able to find the document again. I needed to remember that almost every document can be replicated, so my perfectionism was misplaced. In this case, a wrong decision was better than no decision at all.

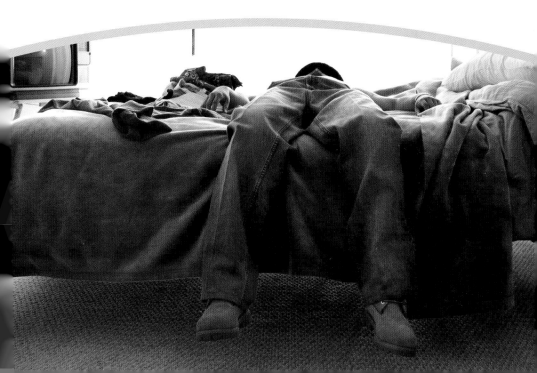

IT MIGHT BE USEFUL SOMEDAY

This is a very common reason why people hang on to stuff. "You never know when it might be needed," they say. This distorted thinking infects my attitude toward e-mails. There are scores of them that have been hanging around my inbox for one to two years. I have been afraid to delete them because the information they contain might be useful in the future. I recognize that now as distorted thinking because if no one needed them in all this time, it is far-fetched to think they ever will.

The "useful someday" perspective also pertains to physical possessions. That perfectly good tie could come back into fashion. That old, beat-up blanket just might come in handy. The space they take up in your closet or garage in anticipation of some unlikely future happening are not worth it.[43] They also take up precious mental and emotional space as well.

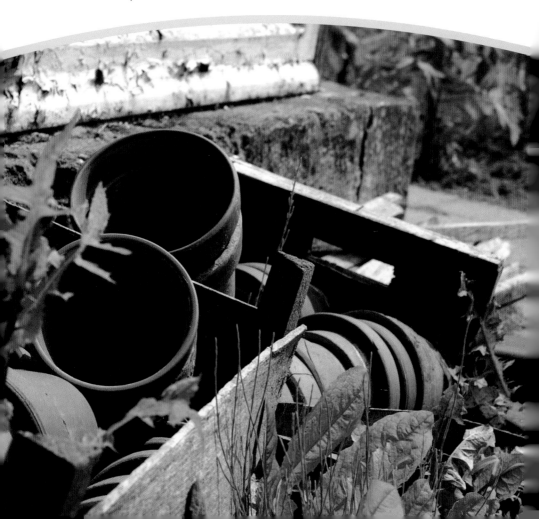

OBLIGATION

Someone hangs onto grandma's black shawl that she gave them ten years ago before she died because they don't want to dishonor her memory by ditching it. They wouldn't be caught dead wearing the thing, but feel obligated to keep it nonetheless. The truth is that grandma would most likely be in favor of you de-cluttering your life. A better way to honor her is through positive memories and by donating the shawl to a local thrift store. You are also letting go of a small bit of guilt.[44]

A sense of obligation can also arise in relation to gifts. We feel that even though we can't stand the thing, the giver would be mortified if they found out that we tossed it. The truth is that they might have given it to you because they didn't want it themselves. Re-gifting. Most of the time people don't remember what they bought for others anyway.

FEAR OF GOING WITHOUT

Individuals who have lived through hard times will sometimes over-purchase for fear of going without again. Instead of one can of soup, they'll buy five. For that same reason they can't resist sales. The opportunity to stock up for less becomes almost irresistible. Every store has some kind of "good deal" all the time so the stuff accumulates. Food gets out of date but hangs around nonetheless instead of being thrown away. It creates a false sense of security.[45]

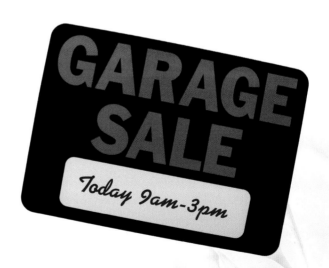

FRUGALITY

A person can't imagine getting rid of that treadmill they never use because they paid so much for it five years ago. The additional emotional price they are paying to keep it around only compounds the problem. Not to mention the space it takes up with boxes piled on top of it. They don't consider that donating it might help someone else. The past is the past. Just because they paid a lot for it years ago is no reason to allow it to impinge on their environment today. It's time to accept that you made a bad decision when you purchased the thing and move on with your life.[46]

All of these rationales and more cause stuff to accumulate that has no direct, positive influence on our lives. Confronting the distorted thinking that is the source of the problem and doing something about it can provide a number of important benefits. It creates more physical space, boosts your energy, frees you from guilt, lowers your stress, increases your peace of mind, makes you more generous, detaches you from your possessions, allows you to have friends over without worrying about being embarrassed, and raises your productivity by no longer having to waste it on managing clutter.[47]

> *The goal is not zero clutter all the time, but reducing it enough so that it doesn't get in your way, physically, emotionally, or spiritually.*

The Gospel of Matthew records the following important counsel from the lips of Jesus, "Do not lay up for yourselves treasures on earth, where moth and rust destroy and where thieves break in and steal; but lay up for yourselves treasures in heaven, where neither moth nor rust destroys and where thieves do not break in and steal" (Matthew 6:19-20, NKJV). Things can become "treasurers" even if they have no particular monetary value. They become valuable to us for a variety of non-monetary reasons. These heart connections, these mental and emotional attachments, can be hard to break, even when those items have lost their usefulness and are simply occupying space.

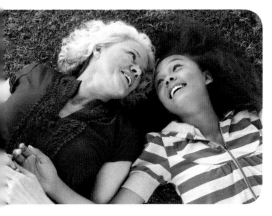

Christ provides us with a perspective that can help loosen our grip. He gives us a powerful perspective by drawing a sharp contrast between the temporary and the eternal. All material things here on earth are destructible, subject to wear and tear. They can be here one day and gone the next. On the other hand, there are *intangible* things that last forever such as love, good deeds, and service. These are impervious to deterioration and have eternal significance. He is trying to help us understand that, ultimately, stuff is only stuff, and we will experience far more satisfaction and joy if we hoard items that make a long lasting impact.

Jesus then delivers the punchline, "For where your treasure is, there your heart will be also" (Matthew 6:21, NKJV). At its root, the issue is our value system. What matters to us the most? What captures our attention and interest the most? Material things are not bad, they simply need to be kept in proper perspective. When that perspective gets distorted, our behavior gets distorted. The key to changing our behavior then, is to change our value system. One of the best ways to stop clinging to the things of this world is to place much more importance on possessing a lifestyle of kindness and caring toward others.

In the New Testament book of Hebrews, the apostle Paul urges us to "throw off everything that hinders" (Heb. 12:1, NIV). We should do that, he says, so that we can "run with perseverance the race marked out for us." Getting rid of clutter enables us to pursue God's path and purpose more effectively. To use another analogy, clutter is like the ropes that hold down a hot air balloon that is made to rise upward. Overcoming clutter is like cutting those ropes, one by one, so we can rise to new heights of spiritual development.

Ecclesiastes tells us that there is: "A time to keep, and a time to throw away" (Eccl. 3:6, NKJV). If you have "hoarder tendencies" like me and are harboring clutter to whatever degree and for whatever reason, consider taking the Bible writer's advice and discover the life-giving environment that God intended.

DISCUSSION

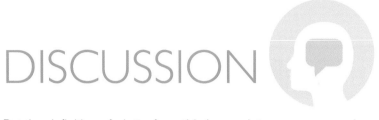

Put the definition of *clutter* from this lesson into your own words.

....

....

Do you or someone you know have "hoarding tendencies" to some degree? Please describe.

....

....

Is it OK for a child to have a messy room? Why or why not?

....

....

How do you relate to clutter emotionally?

....

....

If you taught a class on why it's helpful to de-clutter our homes, what is one of the main points your first lecture would include?

....

....

Tell of a time recently when you struggled with the "it might be useful someday" perspective.

....

....

What awareness from this lesson could help you the most to part with unnecessary things in your environment?

....

....

How might clutter hinder our spiritual growth?

....

....

SHARING

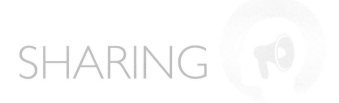

OPPORTUNITY #4:

- Pray for God to open the way for you to share something from these lessons to help someone else this week.

- Keep your radar up each day for opportunities.

ABUNDANT LIVING THOUGHT

Clutter is not really about messiness and disorder. It involves allowing any number of items into our environment that are no longer directly related to our peace, happiness, and sense of well-being.

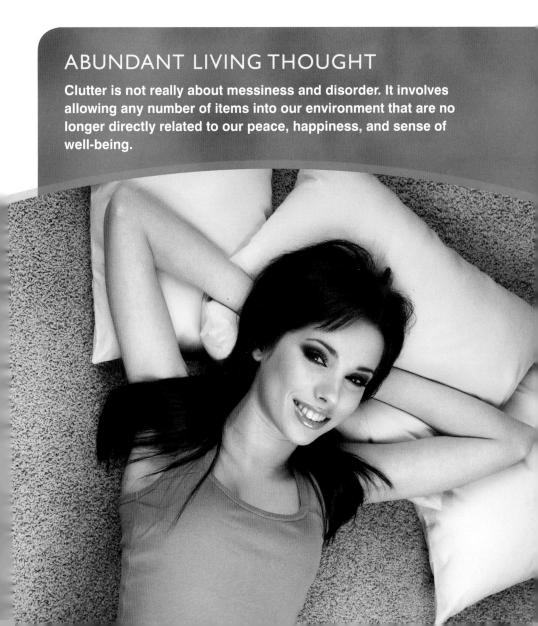

COLORING YOUR WORLD

LESSON FIVE

WARM UP

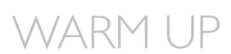

Feedback: In what ways did God open the door last week for you to share some part of the lessons with someone else?

. . . .

. . . .

. . . .

. . . .

Choose one or both questions to discuss (if in group setting)
or write out your answers on a separate sheet (for individual use):

1. **Describe a time when you had loads of fun.**[48]

. . . .

. . . .

. . . .

2. **What color best describes your mood recently?**[49]

. . . .

. . . .

. . . .

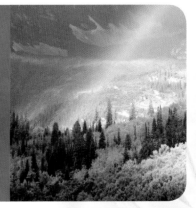

"A man's character always takes its hue, more or less, from the form and color of things about him."

FREDERICK DOUGLASS

DISCOVERY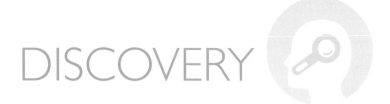

Building a house is only half the battle. You also have to decide how to decorate the interior. My wife and I tend toward subdued colors and natural tones that are easy on the eyes. Tan, soft-yellow, off-white, muted lilac. That was fine for most of the house, but our new abode contained the largest master bedroom we had ever inhabited and we wanted it to be special, out of the ordinary, exceptional. We wanted it to have "character."

My wife and I had just perused several home decorating magazines to get ideas, and the word "bold" kept cropping up. "Make a statement," they said. "Let your adventurous side come out," they urged. Not being particularly adventurous by nature, their challenge was definitely a stretch for us. But we didn't want our new bedroom to look as if it was slept in by interior decorating Neanderthals who were oblivious to the latest trends, so we decided to go bold.

The paint store gave us a series of one inch by one inch cardboard samples of various possibilities. We had heard that strong pinks fostered a romantic mood so we gave that color number to our contractor. Two days later we revisited the house to check out the new décor. First stop, the master bedroom. I entered full of anticipatory delight. Instead I felt like was standing in the belly of a whale that had just downed two hundred gallons of antacid medicine.

I blinked three or four times then looked again. Spread out onto all four walls, the small sample of romantic pink became a *flaming hot pink*, hot enough to incinerate dinner. We quickly repainted to a natural color that was less likely to cause us to go crazy.

Color is one of the strongest influencers in our environment. We often take it for granted, but are affected by it nonetheless. If we want to create life-giving surroundings, one of the best things we can do is to intentionally choose the colors we want to envelope us at home and, if possible, at work.

Colors can encourage relaxation or stimulate activity. They strongly impact our emotions, evoking memories and creating moods, from calmness to anxiety. They play tricks with our perception, making rooms appear larger or smaller. They tell a story about the inhabitants' personality and preferences.[50]

One of the more startling scientific facts that I have encountered is that nothing around us inherently has color. My wife still rebels at the idea, but it is nonetheless true. What we perceive as an object's color is simply the portion of light that it reflects back to our eyeball.

Light from the sun is made up of the combination of all colors. When sunlight hits an object, some of the colors are absorbed and some of them bounce off. A white object reflects back all of the colors. A black object reflects back practically none. So that luscious, ripe tomato that seems deliciously red, is not intrinsically red at all. It is simply absorbing all the colors *except red,* which is reflected back to the retina in our eyes.[51]

Each color is a different wavelength of light. These wavelengths are so small that they have to be measured in *nano*meters (nm). Each nanometer is one *billionth* of a meter long. The wavelength of visible violet ranges from 400-436 nanometers; blue is 436-495 nm; green 495-566 nm; yellow 566-589 nm; orange 589-627 nm; and visible red 627-700 nm.[52] Therefore violet and blue are the shortest wavelengths we can see and red is the longest. Amazingly, we can discern variations in color of as little as 2 nanometers![53]

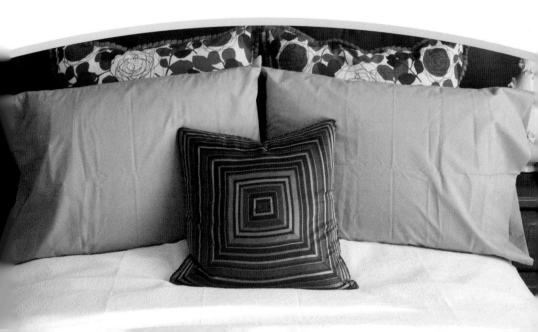

Our eyes are exquisitely designed by God to receive the wavelengths that come our way, then convert them to electrical signals and send them up the optic nerve to the brain. Almost magically, our brain then interprets each type of electrical signal as a different color. So vision actually happens in our *brains*, not in our eyes.

The inside of the human eye is a marvel to behold. Having two of them is a precious possession. The retina at the back of the eye has photoreceptor cells called "rods" that do not perceive color but enable us to see blacks and grays in dim light. There are about 120 million in each eye. We also have six million other photoreceptor cells called "cones" that have the incredible ability to transform wavelengths into color.[54]

Just imagine what our life would be like if our eyes had no cones – everything would be simply various shades of gray. Suppose you went shopping for new clothes and the choices were dark gray, light gray, muted gray, brilliant gray, loud gray, soft gray, charcoal gray, ash gray, gravestone gray, greyhound gray, etc. Terrible.

There are certain wavelengths of light that we cannot perceive such as ultra-violet and infra-red. They are invisible to us. We are restricted to only a certain portion of the light spectrum. But that still leaves an astonishing number of colors to brighten our world. We can, in fact, distinguish millions of different color variations.[55]

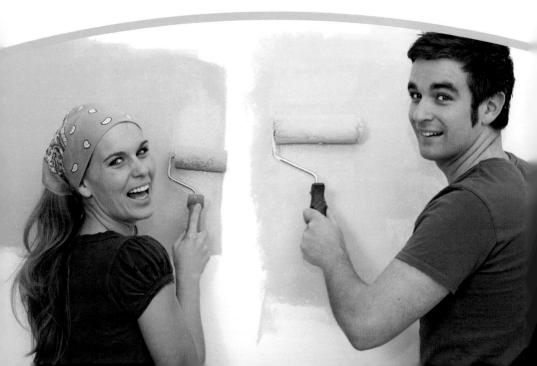

Sunsets are one of the most spectacular light shows we have the privilege of witnessing on a regular basis. They are painted in such blazing colors because of what happens to various wavelengths as the earth turns. At the end of the day when the sun gets closer to the horizon, the sunbeams have to travel through more of earth's atmosphere to get to our eyes. The atmosphere contains numerous particles and the sunbeams hit so many of them at sunset that the shorter wavelengths like violet and blue get blocked out. Other colors with longer wavelengths, like red and orange, are able to survive the journey and mix together in fantastic ways to fill the sky with fire-like hues.[56]

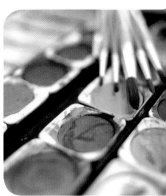

Light has three *primary* colors – *red, yellow, and blue.* They are called primary because you cannot make them from combining any other colors. All other colors are made from these three. When you mix two primary colors together you get what are called *secondary* colors:

Red + yellow = orange

Yellow + blue = green

Blue + red = purple

By varying the shades and intensity of the primary colors, you can produce a wide variety of secondary colors. The secondary colors are then mixed to produce yet another category. On and on it goes, mixing and matching, seemingly forever.[57]

Blues, greens, and purples are known as "cool" colors because they have relaxing, calming effects. They also make rooms feel larger. Yellows, reds, and oranges are known as "warm" colors because they stimulate a stronger emotional response. They make a room feel smaller and more cozy.[58]

The colors that surround us each day have both a physiological and psychological influence on our lives. They can impact both our bodies and our moods.

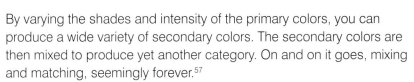

Let's look at a few examples:

Red – In response to the color red, the hormone epinephrine can be released, which causes you to breathe more rapidly. It also increases your blood pressure, heart rate, and the amount of adrenaline in your system.[59] Studies indicate that people associate red with words like passion, strength, activity, excitement, and dignity.[60] It is also known to rev up your appetite and therefore appears in many restaurants to entice you to order.[61] All of a sudden, you get this craving for a sandwich and salad combo and probably never imagined it could be traced back to the color of the walls.

Red is a good choice for a living room or dining room because it can stimulate conversation. Avoid using it in the bedroom, however, where you want something more restful.[62] If my wife and I had gone ahead with hot pink in our bedroom décor, we would have turned into insomniacs.

Blue – We usually perceive lighter blues as calming and soothing. They reduce stress, tension, and high blood pressure and foster concentration.[63] Darker shades of blue, however, can induce melancholy attitudes when used to cover entire walls. People unknowingly refer to that fact when they say things like, "I've got the blues." Because of its connection with sky and water, blue can enhance our feeling of security and constancy. Blue is also the color of winners, who take home blue ribbons.

Yellow – Because of its association with the sun, yellow evokes feelings of happiness, creativity, imagination, energy, cheerfulness, and joy. It is not by accident that the smiley face symbol we see so often is colored yellow. I just painted my den a shade of yellow that helps elevate my mood.

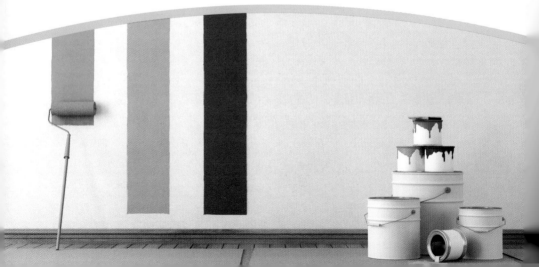

Green – The color green brings to mind scenes of nature, from grass to leaves. It has the connotation of life and hope as the first color we look for in spring. It is the most restful color for the eyes. Located between blue and yellow, it becomes more stimulating when it tends toward yellow and more refreshing and relaxing when it leans toward blue.[64] Bringing green plants into the home creates an uplifting environment.

Orange – In terms of its ability to stimulate and attract attention, orange is perceived as the hottest of all colors, sometimes quite literally. In an air-conditioned factory that had light blue walls, the employees complained about feeling cold even though the thermostat was set at a toasty 75 degrees. Someone who knew their colors repainted the walls orange, and the employees now thought that 75 degrees was too hot and asked that the temperature be turned down to 72![65]

Along with red and yellow, orange stimulates our appetite. It has connotations of being playful, gregarious, glowing, jovial, and cheerful.[66]

Purple – Lighter versions of purple such as lavender and lilac can be calming and restful. Word associations with purple include rich, dramatic, sophisticated, and luxurious.[67] Tyrian purple, the color of the Roman Emperor's toga, was made from shellfish. When crushed, each shellfish yielded about one drop of a whitish liquid. When enough was collected, the cloth was saturated and left to dry in the sunlight where it eventually turned a deep, reddish-purple, like the color of eggplant.[68]

One of the most stunning displays of color in the entire universe is at the throne of God, as described by the apostle John in the book of Revelation: "And the one who sat there had the appearance of jasper and ruby. A rainbow that shone like an emerald encircled the throne. Surrounding the throne were twenty-four other thrones, and seated on them were twenty-four elders. They were dressed in white and had crowns of gold on their heads. From the throne came flashes of lightning, rumblings and peals of thunder. In front of the throne, seven lamps were blazing… Also in front of the throne there was what looked like a sea of glass, clear as crystal" (Rev. 4:2-6, NIV).

It's no wonder that the beings around the throne were so captivated that they cried out,

> *"You are worthy, our Lord and God, to receive glory and honor and power, for you created all things, and by your will they were created and have their being" (Rev. 4:11, NIV).*

DISCUSSION

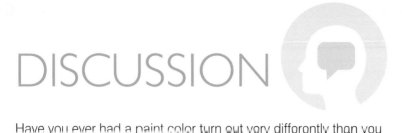

Have you ever had a paint color turn out very differently than you expected after it was applied? What happened?

....

....

Does it change your view of the environment at all to know that nothing has color in and of itself?

....

....

Describe one of the colors you find *relaxing*. Why does it have that effect on you?

....

....

Describe a color you find most *energizing*. Where do you see it?

....

....

Would you eat perfectly good mashed potatoes in a restaurant if they were intentionally colored purple using a safe food coloring? Why or why not?

....

....

What color best captures your mood at present?

....

....

Imagine a color in your mind and try to get others to guess what it is by describing it without using the names of any colors.

....

....

You are standing before the throne of God. What specific thing catches your attention besides God himself? Describe the throne's color.

....

....

....

SHARING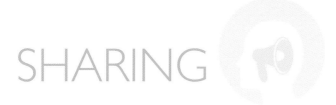

OPPORTUNITY #5:

- Pray for God to open the way for you to share something from these lessons to help someone else this week.

- Keep your radar up each day for opportunities.

ABUNDANT LIVING THOUGHT

If we want to create life-giving surroundings, one of the best things we can do is to intentionally choose the colors we want to envelope us at home and, if possible, at work.

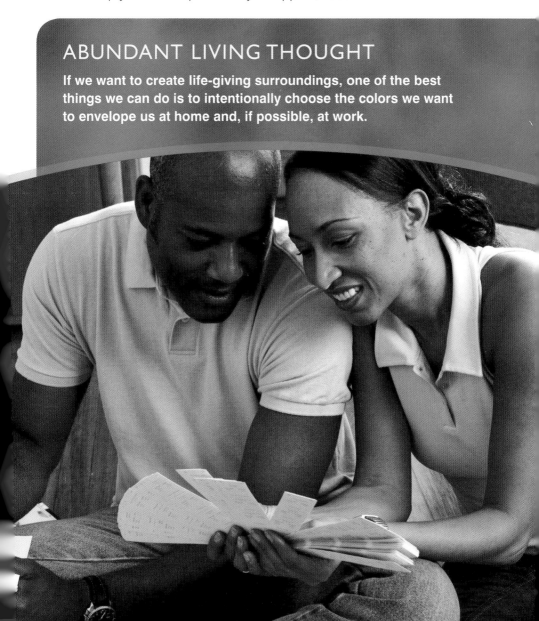

SOUNDS OF LIFE

LESSON SIX

WARM UP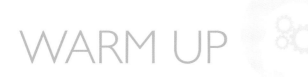

Feedback: In what ways did God open the door last week for you to share some part of the lesson with someone else?

....

....

....

....

Choose one or both questions to discuss (if in group setting)
or write out your answers on a separate sheet (for individual use):

1. **"What do you wish people would ask you about?"**[69]

....

....

....

....

2. **"What is something you wish you never had to worry about again?"**[70]

....

....

....

....

> *"Imagine sitting quietly in the middle of God's garden with only the sounds of nature filling your ears and calming your spirit: birds chirping, a brook flowing, the breeze gently rustling leaves."*
>
> **DES CUMMINGS JR., PhD**

DISCOVERY

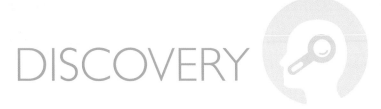

My wife, daughter, and I approached the concert hall with a growing sense of excitement. We had tickets to hear a legend from my childhood. During the drive there, I had replayed the performer's chart-topping songs from way back in the 1960s. They were easy-listening folk songs similar to those sung by Peter, Paul, and Mary or Simon and Garfunkel – gentle tunes with simple melodies and deeply meaningful words about life, love, joy, and sadness. I relished the opportunity to hear them played again live.

On the inside, the concert hall looked like a half-sized basketball stadium. Our last-minute tickets put us as high up and as far back from the stage as you could get without being on the other side of the exit door. No problem, at least we were in. After getting oriented, I felt bad for the hundreds of people who filled the main floor but had nowhere to sit. I asked the young man next to me about it and he assured me it was very normal at concerts like this.

His "like this" caught my attention. I had only known one kind of concert – musicians performing and listeners sitting in neatly laid out, numbered seats. Was there some *other* kind? Obviously yes. The seat-less people were laughing, chatting, and milling around, clearly pleased with their situation.

The band eventually came on stage to raucous cheers and applause. I leaned forward in anticipation, elbows on knees, chin in my hands. The guitars hit the first chord. Honestly, it was so loud I thought a bomb had gone off. As the music continued, the sound waves were like a wind forcing me backward. I could feel the pressure on my chest. In order to be heard, I had to shout at my wife who sat right next to me. She yelled back something I couldn't understand. So much for folksy melodies from the 60s. The legend had obviously re-invented himself.

I could only make out an occasional word in the lyrics. A typical verse came across to me as: "___ ___ ___ ___ ___ ___ cars ___ ___ ___ ___ now!" Sometimes I would pick up two or three words in a row, which helped immensely in trying to piece together the theme. We left early and could still hear the band when we arrived at our car thirty-five parking lot rows away.

That's one noisy end of the sound spectrum. The other end is the many days my wife and I have kayaked down rivers and stopped paddling to listen to the subtle sounds of nature. We have to be patient, attentive, and quiet, but are almost always deeply rewarded by hearing:

- Bullfrogs exchanging base notes.
- Male crickets chirping by rubbing their wings together at dusk.
- Blue herons scolding.
- Fish leaping up and splashing back.
- Impatient crows squawking.
- Duck feet slapping the water to get above the surface for take-off.
- Bees busily buzzing.
- The faint crow of a rooster somewhere in the distance.
- Water bubbling in our wake.
- Wind fingering the leaves.

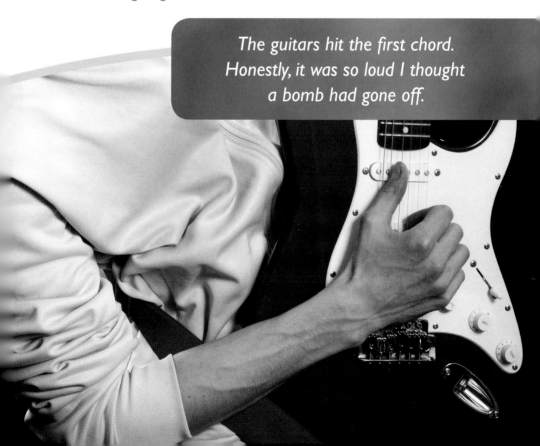

The guitars hit the first chord. Honestly, it was so loud I thought a bomb had gone off.

Sound is one of the most prominent features of our environment. The world is full of all kinds of sounds, from wondrous to annoying, and it is our enormous privilege to be able to hear them, even the annoying ones.

Nothing has made me more aware of the sounds around me than taking time to learn the rudiments of how the human ear works. As I began to comprehend the complex process of hearing, I developed a much deeper appreciation for what it takes to accurately perceive the countless sounds in our multi-faceted world.

The ear is made up of three sections: the outer ear, middle ear, and inner ear, all sealed off from each other by specialized membranes. To grasp the basics of hearing, let's pretend that we are cave explorers walking through a giant ear, poking around with headlamps and an assortment of tools.

We start at the outside of the ear, checking out the flaps of skin and ridges that stick out from either side of the head. Officially called the pinna, they each serve to gather sounds and steer them inside.[71] Sound is basically waves of air particles. These air waves enter our ears just like waves of water ripple across a pond. The pinna of our imaginary ears are over forty feet high.

As explorers, we turn our headlamps on and walk inside the dark corridor of the ear canal to see where the air waves go. After a few steps, we run into small patches of brownish wax that catch pollutants, harden up, then break off and tumble out during sleep or vigorous activity.

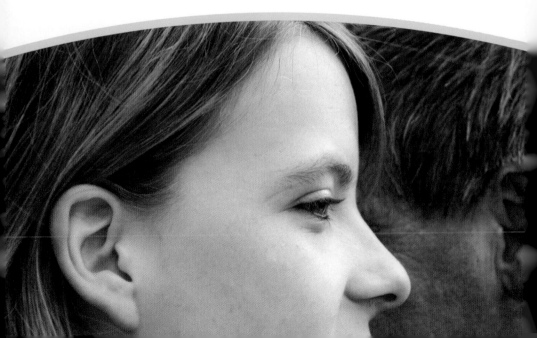

Further on, we encounter a fleshy membrane that completely seals off the way forward. It's the eardrum that vibrates back and forth with every wave of air particles that comes from the outside. *Higher pitched* sound waves cause the eardrum to move more rapidly. *Louder* sounds cause it to move a greater distance.[72]

With no other recourse, you cut a hole near the bottom of the eardrum wall and everyone steps through it. We shine our lamp around the large room in front of us called the middle ear. Above are the three tiniest bones in the body called the hammer, anvil, and stirrup, all linked together. The hammer is attached to the backside of the eardrum and moves with it, which in turns moves the anvil and the stirrup. Across the room, we see that the stirrup is connected to another wall on the other side.[73]

We shine the lamp across the hammer, anvil, and stirrup, carefully examining their exquisite design and linkage. They work like levers. Their purpose is to magnify the intensity of the vibrations coming from the eardrum over twenty times.[74] They need to do that in order to create waves in the hard-to-move fluid inside the cochlea, located in the next sealed chamber called the inner ear.[75]

Everyone uses ropes and ladders to cross the cavernous middle ear. Then someone bores through the next wall, called the oval window, to access the third chamber, the inner ear. Inside, as our eyes adjust, we see the cochlea looming before us with its characteristic snail-like shape. It contains spiraled tubes full of specialized fluid.[76]

We drill a yard wide hole in one of the tubes for us to fit through. We put on our scuba gear and masks, drop into the fluid, and start swimming the long, narrow passageway like traveling in an underwater cave.

Inside the cochlea are little hair-like projections. These biological marvels are each designed to respond to only certain wave frequencies. Higher pitched frequencies set the shorter hairs in motion while lower pitched frequencies move the longer ones further in.[77] These hairs are so sensitive that they respond even when the tip has been moved no more than the width of an atom! That's equivalent to moving the Eiffel Tower only half an inch.[78] The highest frequencies cause them to move back and forth 20,000 times per second![79]

When we lose a portion of our hearing, it is often because some of these delicate hairs have been damaged. Once damaged, they don't grow back.[80] The loudness of a sound is measured in units called decibels. Sounds 75 decibels and below do not cause any damage, but anything above 85 decibels can harm these fine hair structures over time.

Normal conversation is 60-70 dB, a subway train 90 dB, and a rock concert 115 dB.[81] The way the scale works, every increase of 10 dB is actually a tenfold increase in sound energy. Therefore 90 dB is ten times noisier than 80dB.[82] If you have to shout to be heard, your environment is too loud.

As explorer-divers, we are awed to watch the tiny cell hairs move inside the cochlea, sending small electrical signals to the auditory nerve that winds its way over to the brain. Our mind has the extraordinary ability to take all of these nerve signals, sort them out, and reproduce the sound that originally entered the outer ear only a very short time ago. Not only that, but it also connects that sound to memories and emotions to give us a more expansive experience.

It is hard to imagine how all these different elements of the hearing process are able to capture both a baby's whimper in a nearby bedroom and the many complexities of an orchestra playing Mozart's Symphony No. 40 in G minor! It's truly a privilege to possess such an extraordinary organ.

The next time you listen to a piece of music or hear a lecture, think of the air waves traveling into your outer ear, thumping on the eardrum, causing the three tiny bones of the middle ear to vibrate, which, in turn, makes thousands of hair cells pulsate inside the cochlea, an organ no bigger than a pea.[83]

Knowing how complex our hearing mechanism is, we should honor this amazing gift from God by seeking out new sounds on a regular basis and relishing what we discover. To not use our exquisite ears to tune in to more of life's abundant sounds would be like owning a race car and only driving it at 15 miles per hour.

Once you have come to appreciate the ability to hear, you can turn your attention to what kinds of sounds are most helpful to your health and well-being. *Music is probably the most impactful sound of all.*

David was one of the most prominent musicians of the Old Testament Scriptures. He wrote scores of psalms, which were originally designed to be sung. They include many verses that inspire, encourage, comfort, and uplift. When King Saul felt depressed, he called David in to play the lyre, an ancient instrument much like a hand-held harp or guitar. The Scriptures tell us that after listening to the beautiful music, "Saul would become refreshed and well, and the distressing spirit would depart from him" (1 Sam 16:23, NKJV).

We are also told that the Israelite temple utilized an orchestra and choir to create a worshipful atmosphere and put the congregation in touch with God. It contained singers, stringed instruments, cymbals, horns, trumpets, and flutes, with a man named Chenaniah as music director (see 1 Chron. 15:16-29; Psalms 150).

In the New Testament, the apostle Paul must have valued music because he wrote the following to the church in Colossae, "Let the word of Christ dwell in you richly in all wisdom, teaching and admonishing one another in psalms and hymns and spiritual songs, singing with grace in your hearts to the Lord" (Col. 3:17, NKJV).

Turn your attention to what kinds of sounds are most helpful to your health and well-being.

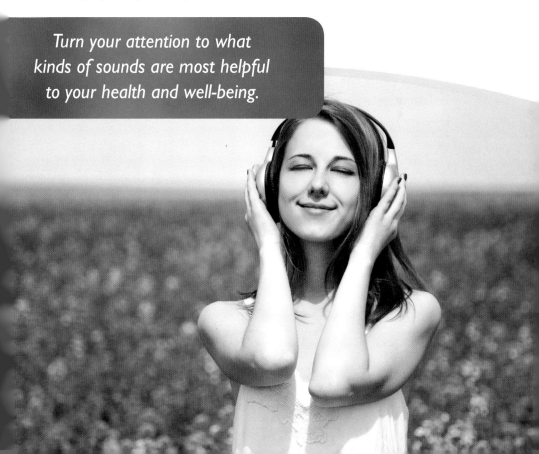

Music can have a similar positive effect on us today. Music occupies more areas of the brain than language does:[84]

1. **Spiritual music can dramatically deepen our relationship with God and open our hearts to the blessings he longs to bestow.**

2. **Listening to music daily can reduce chronic pain by up to 21 percent. It also makes people feel more in control of their pain.[85]**

3. **Music can increase blood flow, reduce stress and anxiety, lower heart rate and blood pressure, improve breathing patterns, boost the immune system, and create an overall feeling of well-being.[86]**

4. **Pleasant music increases the level of dopamine in the brain, a chemical responsible for transmitting signals between nerve cells and fostering a positive mood. Sad songs can also make us feel good by the release of the comfort hormone prolactin in the brain.[87]**

5. **Playing an instrument or singing in a group fosters social connections and support.**

6. **Listening to music while exercising decreases boredom and increases endurance.[88]**

7. **Taking music lessons can enhance IQ and SAT scores.[89]**

8. **Office workers who were able to listen to their favorite music found it soothed frayed nerves, drowned out distracting office noise, boosted mood, and also improved performance.[90]**

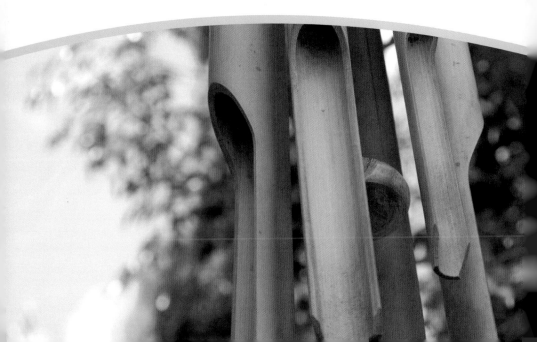

Jesus had some very important things to say about our use of the gift of hearing. For instance, he commended Mary when she took time away from her chores to listen carefully to his words (Luke 10:39). Mary's sister Martha got hot under the collar because she felt dumped on, but as far as Christ was concerned the chores could wait. This was a "teaching moment" that superseded dinner preparation. The lesson for us today is to make sure we are taking adequate time for spiritual listening and to not let the voice of the Master get crowded out by the press of our daily tasks.

At another time, Christ also said, "My sheep hear my voice, and I know them, and they follow me" (John 10:27). Sheep could distinguish between the call of their own shepherd and that of some other sheepherder. Their leader's voice had a distinctive timber and resonance they could trust. It was a voice that meant safety and nourishment. They had heard that voice since they were little lambs and knew it well.

Likewise, the more time we spend listening to what Jesus has to say in Scripture, the more we will be able recognize whether or not our own thoughts and the thoughts of others are consistent with what we have been hearing from him.

Jesus also commended the wisdom of those who not only heard him but also applied his teachings to their lives. "Therefore whoever hears these sayings of mine, *and does them,* I will liken him to a wise man who built his house on the rock" (Matthew 7:24). When the floods come, the house stands, because it has a solid foundation. The only way to build that kind of strong foundation in our own lives is to not only know what is best but to also incorporate those teachings and values into our daily lives. We may do so very imperfectly, but Jesus honors the desires and intensions of our hearts.

The ability to hear is a marvel of engineering from the hand of our Creator. It was given from his heart of love to enable us to experience life to the fullest.

DISCUSSION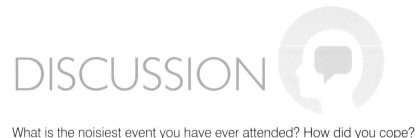

What is the noisiest event you have ever attended? How did you cope?

....

....

What is one of the sounds you recollect from childhood?

....

....

What fact about how we hear stood out in your mind from the lesson?

....

....

What is one of your favorite sounds other than music? Duplicate the sound now as best you can.

....

....

Describe a brand new sound you have heard in the last two months.

....

....

What is one of the sounds you would miss the most if you could not hear (other than hearing someone's voice)?

....

....

Describe the sound of Jesus' voice as you imagine it.

....

....

Which of the following captures how your week has been going? Why?

SURF

....

WIND CHIMES

....

DRUMS

....

VIOLIN

....

TRAFFIC

....

SHARING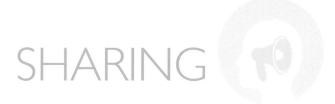

OPPORTUNITY #6:

- Pray for God to open the way for you to share something from these lessons to help someone else this week.

- Keep your radar up each day for opportunities.

ABUNDANT LIVING THOUGHT

Knowing how complex our hearing mechanism is, we should honor this amazing gift from God by seeking out new sounds on a regular basis and relishing what we discover.

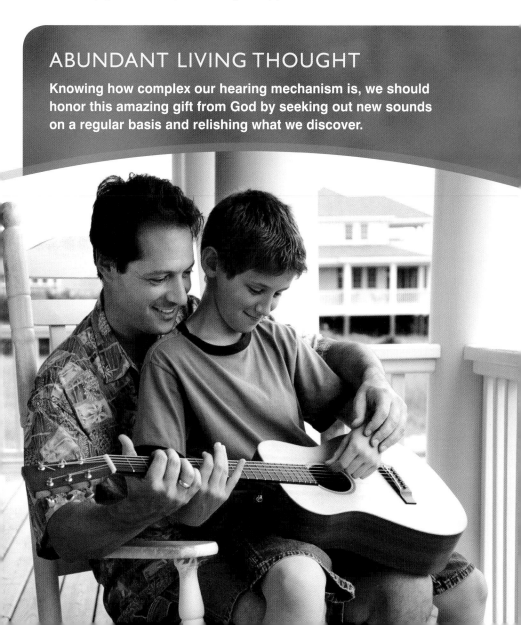

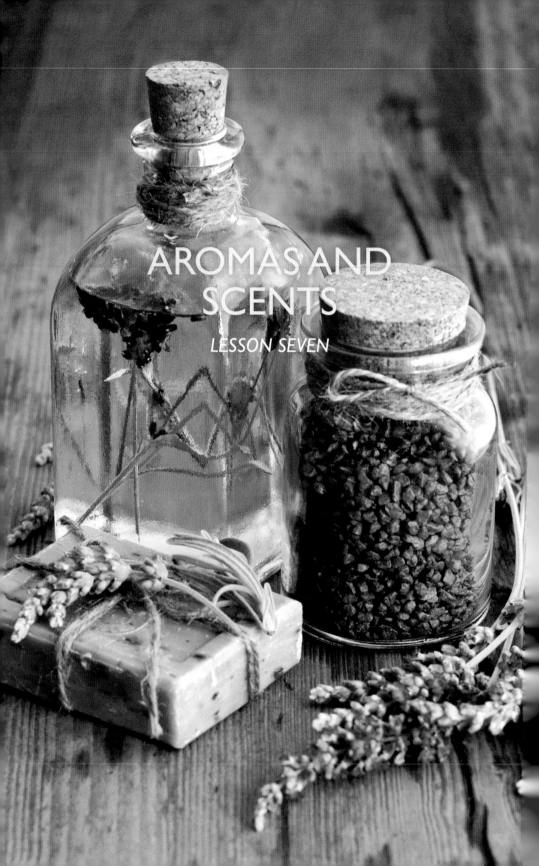

AROMAS AND SCENTS

LESSON SEVEN

WARM UP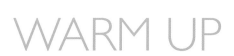

Feedback: In what ways did God open the door last week for you to share some part of the lessons with someone else?

....

....

....

....

Choose one or both questions to discuss (if in group setting) or write out your answers on a separate sheet (for individual use):

1. **What song evokes a special response from you whenever you hear it? Why?**

....

....

....

....

2. **"What's missing in your life?"**[91]

....

....

....

....

> *"Scents associated with natural things — flowers, fresh air, the sea — tend to have a soothing affect on most people because those aromas take them... to a garden, a mountain retreat, or a beautiful beach."*
>
> **DR. DICK TIBBITS**

DISCOVERY

My fellow staff member Mike and I were great friends and we loved to play practical jokes on each other. I thought my newest idea had real potential.

One summer evening, I purchased a whole dead fish about a foot long and kept it wrapped out in my garage overnight. The next morning I put the fish in a bag and left for work quite early. At the office, I walked into Mike's office, unwrapped the carcass, and gleefully taped it under his desk chair. The fish already smelled, and I was sure that by the time he arrived, his office would be quite odiferous.

Most likely, Mike would discover the source of the odor rather quickly and get rid of the offending fish, but at least he'd have to endure the leftover smell for an hour or so.

My friend walked in at 8:30 a.m. By 9:30 a.m., he hadn't said anything.

By 10:00 a.m., I was bursting with curiosity, so I strolled nonchalantly through his office to catch a whiff. It smelled fishy alright, worse than I expected. Instead of dissipating, the smell had actually intensified. As I passed by, Mike smiled and continued processing paper work.

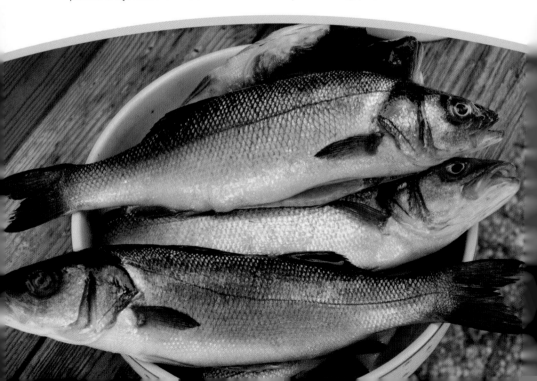

"What's going on?" I wondered.

At 11:00 a.m., the Workers Compensation auditor arrived unexpectedly at Mike's office for his periodic review. He used a spare desk, off to one corner. By noon he was done. "Poor guy," I thought as he hurried out the side entrance with a white hanky over his face.

My sense of wonder and amusement grew as the day progressed. By mid-afternoon, Mike's office smelled like a fishing dock.

At about thirty minutes to closing, Mike suddenly got up and headed out of the office. On the way out, he popped his head in my door and casually said, "Hey Kim, I'm leaving a little early today. I picked up a really bad head cold last night and my nose is all stuffed up. See you tomorrow." He couldn't smell a thing.

Disappointed, I retrieved the fish and threw it in the outside dumpster. Even today, the right odor at the Supermarket Seafood Department can take me back all those years as if it was yesterday – the office, the chair, the fish, the duct tape, the auditor.

Smell is a very powerful sense. It is a wonderful gift from God that will hopefully enable us to experience many more uplifting odors than repulsive ones.

The ability to smell is one of the key ways that we are able to engage our environment. Understanding the basics of how the sense of smell works can help us appreciate it more deeply and inspire us to use it more extensively to explore the wide spectrum of aromas in our world.

Our noses are designed as multi-purpose organs. They warm and moisten air that we inhale. They also clean up dirt, dust, pollen, and other unwanted items (even the occasional bug) by use of nose hairs lining the inner walls. This "trash" is then mingled with mucus and moved further up the nose by cells that act like tiny brooms. Eventually, everything drips down the back of our throat where much of it is swallowed.[92]

Noses are also, of course, able to smell and detect odors and scents. They are thousands of times more sensitive than our other senses.[93] What we smell are the molecules that come from things around us. Roses emit molecules. Oranges emit molecules. Perfume and aftershave give off molecules. People emit odor molecules. They become airborne and some of them drift into our nostrils as we inhale. Once trapped inside, they make their way into the upper reaches of our nasal passages. Many odors are not single molecules, but a mixture.[94]

The odor molecules eventually enter a large cavern where a postage stamp sized area is packed with millions of nerve cells called *olfactory receptors*. In 2004, a Nobel Prize was awarded to two scientists, Richard Axel and Linda Buck, who had figured out that these receptors each specialize in particular odors. The receptors wait patiently until the right type of odor molecules come their way. When that happens, the molecules and receptors connect together perfectly like putting the right key into the right lock.[95]

Columbia University Medical Center Executive Vice President Gerald D. Fischbach commented on the work of Axel and Buck, saying that their findings are "among the most important studies of the past fifty years, providing insights regarding how individuals perceive their external environment."[96] Scientists are now also able to identify where many scent molecules will fall on a type of "pleasantness scale" according to their molecular structure.[97]

Once connected to their preferred molecules, the receptors send an electrical signal to the brain. It is up to the brain to recognize each type of signal and conclude that, for instance, "Those must be molecules from an orange." Our incredible brains can distinguish many different scents according to which types of electrical signals are being sent its way![98]

The odor signal travels to a part of the brain that also deals with emotions, memories, and learning. A big part of how we recognize different smells relates to how we associate them with different memories and events. Just before we put the first orange slice we ever ate into our mouth, our nose got a whiff and forever matches what it smelled with what our eyes saw and what we tasted. We also remember whether the experience felt pleasurable or not. The linkage to memory is why certain smells today can evoke memories of events that happened many years ago.

The connection between smells and emotion is why aromas can also significantly affect our moods.[99] It is a linkage that advertisers love to exploit. For example, real estate agents may tell a home owner to have cookies baking in the oven during an open house. Many marketing companies try to figure out how smells can motivate us to buy everything from food to clothing. One savvy pastor used the smell-mood connection to make a sermon illustration come alive. As he spoke about popcorn, someone directed the odor of freshly cooked popcorn into the ventilation system where it then wafted over the delighted congregation.

Our noses are true marvels of heavenly design. Understanding and appreciating their intricacy can help us become more conscious of the aromas around us and can also motivate us to make better use of our noses to proactively seek out and experience new smells. We could even take our own "Aroma Safaris."

The connection between smells and emotion is why aromas can also significantly affect our moods.

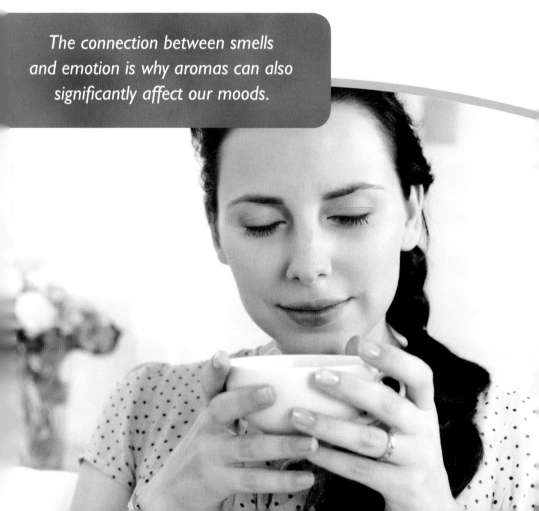

The Scriptures have much to say about aromas. One of the most aromatic chapters in the Bible is found in Exodus 30 where God provides the recipe for oil to anoint the Old Testament Sanctuary and for incense to be burned on an altar.

The Oil – God spoke to Moses: "Take the best spices: twelve and a half pounds of liquid myrrh; half that much, six and a quarter pounds, of fragrant cinnamon; six and a quarter pounds of fragrant cane; twelve and a half pounds of cassia... and a gallon of olive oil. Make these into a holy anointing oil, a perfumer's skillful blend" (Exodus 30:22-25, The Message).

God certainly loves fragrant smells!
No wonder he gave us
noses in order to share the joy.

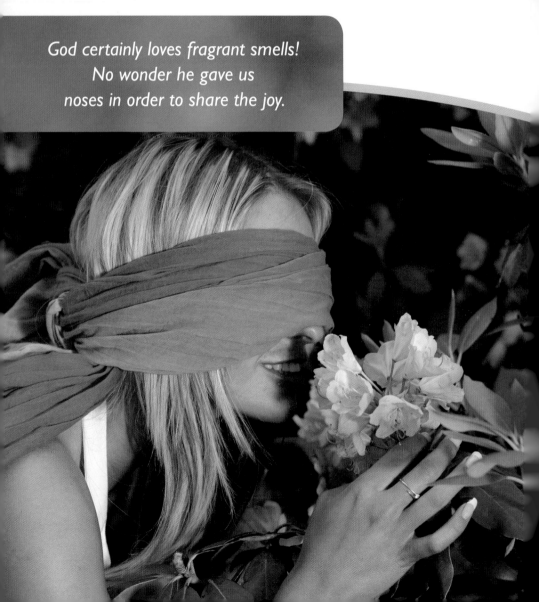

The Incense – GOD spoke to Moses: "Take fragrant spices – gum resin, onycha, galbanum – and add pure frankincense. Mix the spices in equal proportions to make an aromatic incense" (Exodus 30: 34-35, The Message).

God certainly loves fragrant smells! No wonder he gave us noses in order to share the joy. The Bible also talks about other aromatics as well, such as hyssop and spikenard ointment.

I love the passage in Ezekiel 20:41 where God compares his followers to a very pleasant smell. He says, "I will accept you as a sweet aroma." He is essentially saying, "When I think of you, it will remind me of the sweetest of aromas, like a lovely rose."

In New Testament times, when the apostle Paul sent a letter to the church members in the city of Philippi, he compared their generosity to a marvelous fragrance: "And now I have it all – and keep getting more! The gifts you sent with Epaphroditus were more than enough, like a sweet-smelling sacrifice roasting on the altar, filling the air with fragrance, pleasing God no end" (Phil. 4:18, The Message).

In the last book of the Bible, Revelation, people's prayers are compared to bowls full of incense. Our prayers are one of God's favorite aromas.

God also gave us some aromas to help with our health and well-being. According to Theresa Molnar, executive director of the Sense of Smell Institute in New York City, "Scents can have positive effects on mood, stress reduction, sleep enhancement, self-confidence, and physical and cognitive performance."[100]

Australian psychologist John Prescott indicates that because of the mind-body connection, smell can improve pain tolerance. He says that, "Any pleasant smell can act as a distraction and lift mood, but recent studies suggest that sweet smells might work best."[101]

Since smells can be so enjoyable and uplifting, we would do well to explore how they might be deployed in our homes and workplaces more effectively. The following is a list of ways that you turn your environment into an aroma haven:

1. Use scented candles.

2. Add scented oil to humidifiers.

3. Display flowers in vases.

4. Hang up bunches of flowers or herbs.

    Jill Blake advises people to, "Hang sweet-smelling flowers or bunches of herbs in the kitchen or dining room. Bay leaves, rosemary, sage, lavender and bergamot smell particularly wonderful. Hang dried herbs in cupboards."[102]

5. Fill dishes with potpourri that includes items like dried rose petals, violets, jasmine, lily of the valley, marigolds, larkspur, pinks, sage, rosemary, bergamot, lavender, lemon verbena, and chamomile. You can also add aromatic herbs, spices, wood shavings, pine cones, cinnamon sticks, plus other great smelling elements to scent the air.[103]

6. Utilize scent warmers or reed diffusers. Reed diffusers are a certain kind of reed with one end in an aromatic oil and the other sticking up out of a container. They require no flame.[104]

7. Grow an indoor herb garden and raise pleasant smelling house plants.

8. Boil herbs to release wonderful scents. Boil water in a pan, then remove from heat. Add a few whole cinnamon sticks, whole cloves, and a small amount of nutmeg. Add fragrant oils as desired. Skins from citrus fruits also work well.[105]

9. Burn incense.

10. Display soaps in a basket.

11. Dilute fragrant oil with water and spray around your home.[106]

12. Air out the house and let nature's aromas in.

Every person I know loves the aroma of chocolate. The science of "sensomics" has broken down that intoxicating smell into its various chemical components. It turns out that the aroma we know as chocolate is made up of a combination of substances that individually smell like potato chips, cooked meat, peaches, raw beef fat, cooked cabbage, human sweat, earth, cucumber, and honey.[107] Put them all together and our brain says, "Chocolate!" Our mind works that kind of magic with other smells as well.

The more we know about the God-given gift of smell, the more we are able to appreciate it and use it gladly to inhale the wonderful aromas in our environment that can be every bit as delightful as the heady scent of chocolate itself.

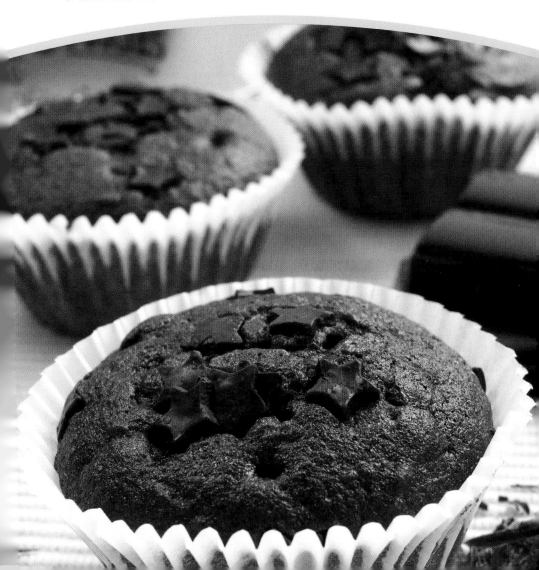

DISCUSSION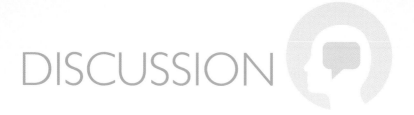

Describe a memorable aroma from your childhood. Why do you think it lingers in your memory?

....
....

Do you take time to absorb the aroma of food before you eat it? What is your favorite?

....
....

What smells do you find relaxing? What other aromas affect your moods? How?

....
....

Which one of the following smells comes the closest to representing how you have been feeling lately? Why?

LAVENDER ....

VANILLA ....

ORANGE SLICES ....

BURNT TOAST ....

STALE BREAD ....

GYM LOCKER ....

What aromas would you miss the most if you were not able to smell?

....
....

Close your eyes for a few moments. What aroma comes to mind from this past week? Why did it stand out?

....
....

What aroma do you think comes to God's mind when he thinks of you?

....
....

....

SHARING

OPPORTUNITY #7:

- Pray for God to open the way for you to share something from these lessons to help someone else this week.

- Keep your radar up each day for opportunities.

ABUNDANT LIVING THOUGHT

We can make better use of our noses to proactively seek out and experience new smells. We could even take our own "Aroma Safaris."

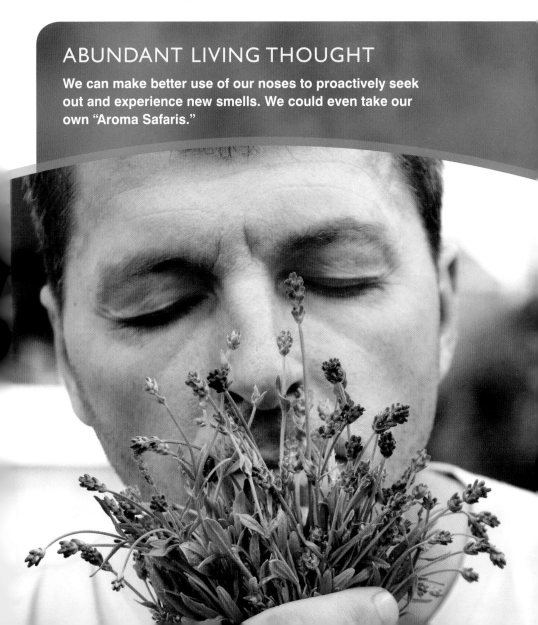

THREE PRECIOUS GIFTS

LESSON EIGHT

WARM UP

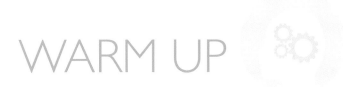

Feedback: In what ways did God open the door last week for you to share some part of the lessons with someone else?

....
....
....
....

Choose one or both questions to discuss (if in group setting) or write out your answers on a separate sheet (for individual use, in which case #1 does not apply):

1. **Share one of your most memorable moments as a member of this group.**

....
....
....

2. **What is one of the biggest "takeaways" you have learned from these lessons? Why is that meaningful for you?**

....
....
....

> *"Nobody can be in good health if he does not have all the time, fresh air, sunshine, and good water."*
>
> **CHIEF FLYING HAWK,
> OGLALA SIOUX**

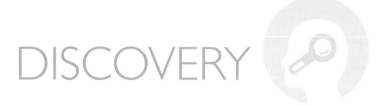

DISCOVERY

PRECIOUS GIFT #1 – WATER

Water is a precious gift that God has provided as part of our environment. We obviously need to drink it, but water can also be used externally to promote health and well-being. It does, however, need to be used properly and my own experience was much less than ideal.

Instead of attending the morning church service with my wife, Ann, I stayed home to nurse a bad cold. Hunkered down in bed, I waited for the over-the-counter medicine to calm my sneezing, coughing, and pounding headache. After a few minutes, I drifted off to a restless sleep.

About 1 p.m., Ann returned, all excited. Someone at church had told her that a hot bath could work wonders. It would ease my symptoms and put me swiftly back on the road to health. A committed shower person, I listened half-heartedly, groaned, and pulled the covers over my head. "It's a waste of time," I grunted.

Not deterred in the least, Ann ripped off the blankets and yanked me to an upright position. "Look," she insisted, "you're going to do this!" I had rarely seen her so jazzed about something. The more I listened, the more convincing she sounded. Still harboring lingering doubts, I decided to go along, if nothing else, to make her stop.

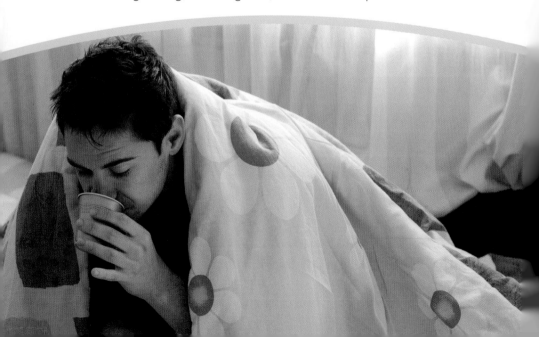

I was soon immersed up to my neck in a hot bath, very hot. As I soaked, the image of a cooked lobster came readily to mind. The water eventually turned more tepid, at which point Ann insisted on draining off a few gallons and adding more steamy water, as hot as I could stand it. Sweat poured off my face. I felt flushed. Another image came to mind of a missionary being stewed in a large pot by starving cannibals.

"Can I get out now?" I begged.

"You need to stay in longer," she replied. Adding softly, "I think." Her eagerness to help had pushed her onto the always treacherous path of, "If a little is good, a lot is better."

Eventually, after about thirty minutes, she told me to stand up. I rose eagerly from within the steam like an apparition and glanced down nervously at my bright red torso. I felt physically drained. After taking my first step out of the tub, I fainted. As Ann informed me later, it wasn't one of those graceful faints like an actress in the movies who puts her arm across her forehead, sighs, and then melts slowly onto the floor. I collapsed in an undignified heap onto the bathroom tile, ashen faced.

Not knowing what else to do, Ann did what she had seen in TV sitcoms. She slapped me several times across the face, desperately trying to bring me around. I awoke groggily. She wanted to call 911. I protested loudly saying, "I can't let them see me like this!" Ann then started dragging me down the hall toward the bedroom. I stopped her, stumbled to my feet, meandered the rest of the way, and slid under the covers. My wife bent over me with a look of great concern and said, "I must have gotten something wrong."

So what should my loving, well-intentioned wife and I have done differently? First, I should have drunk water before and after. Then, the bath temperature should have been tailored to my condition and sensitivity – hot enough to induce a sweat but not too hot, and for only ten to fifteen minutes. Let the bather be the guide. Prior to getting out, cooler water should have been added to bring down my core temperature. When finished, I should have stood up slowly, sat on the edge of the tub until acclimated, and then carefully exited onto a non-slip mat or surface. If a person has a medical condition or illness, consulting a physician is a wise decision in a situation like this.

Hot baths have real benefits, my own misadventure notwithstanding. A properly taken hot bath can:[108]

- Relieve stress, especially when aromatic oils or salts are added.
- Stimulate circulation.
- Foster sleep.
- Assist digestion.
- Help tension headaches.
- Remove toxins.
- Boost the immune system.

Another great external use of water to promote health is a hot *and* cold shower. The following procedure is typical:

Step 1: Turn the shower to warm. Get acclimated. Increase the temperature so that it is comfortably hot. The normal precautions apply if you have a condition or illness. Stay under for 3 minutes.

Step 2: Turn the water as cold as you can stand it for 20-30 seconds. Allow the water to hit the back of your neck first.

Step 3: Turn back to the previous warm temperature for 3 minutes.

Step 4: Return to cold for 20-30 seconds.

Sept 5: Repeat the entire cycle one more time, ending with a few seconds of cold. Step out carefully and wrap yourself in a warm towel or blanket. You can repeat up to three to five cycles if you have time. If cold water is too much for you, use cool.[109]

The beneficial effects of hot/cold showers are similar to many of those from a warm bath. Again, check with your physician to make sure this will indeed benefit you specifically.

Water is a precious gift that God has provided as part of our environment. We obviously need to drink it, but water can also be used externally to promote health and well-being.

PRECIOUS GIFT #2 – FRESH AIR

In 1918 and 1919, a flu pandemic swept across the world causing an estimated twenty to thirty *million* deaths, with over 500,000 deaths in the United States alone. Historical records from the city of Dayton, Ohio dramatically illustrate the disease's impact. It came in three separate waves. The first outbreak in Ohio occurred in September 1918 at a military camp near Chillicothe where eighteen soldiers succumbed during that month. The flu quickly spread outward infecting cities and towns, including Dayton.

Because the flu is an airborne disease, health officials in Dayton eventually closed all public establishments where people gathered together. The ban included schools, churches, theaters, saloons, soda fountains, and pool rooms. Sporting events were frequently cancelled because one or both of the teams could not put enough players on the field. Mourners were discouraged from holding funerals in private homes, which was a common practice at the time. Even funerals held in churches had to be family only.

Thankfully, by the end of 1918, outbreaks dwindled and restrictions on public gatherings were lifted. But tens of thousands had been afflicted and hundreds had perished.

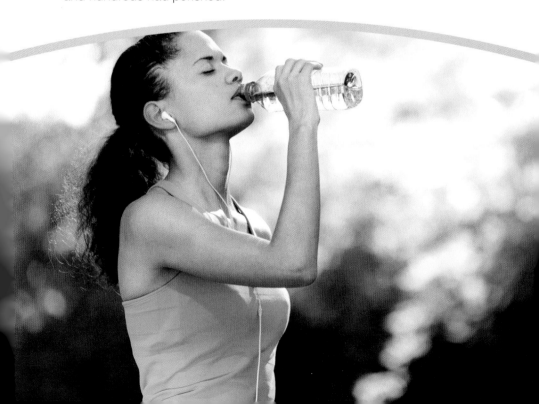

Although there was no medication for the flu at the time, public health officials especially singled out one particular element as being critical for both prevention and cure – *fresh air*. At one point, Dayton's Health Commissioner, Dr. A. O. Peters, issued the following statement, "Custodians of buildings where public gatherings are to be held are requested to see to it that there is plenty of ventilation, without draft, and with a flood of outside air pouring into the building."[110]

Fresh air is one of God's precious gifts to us from our environment. It is vital to our health and well-being and has numerous benefits. We can live only a few short minutes without it. An average person takes about 21,600 breaths each day, so the quality of the air we breathe is a very important consideration.[111]

In order to understand what makes fresh air fresh, I want you to put on some very special glasses, called "*Ion Detectors.*" An ion is simply a molecule that has either a positive or negative charge. We cannot see them, but the air around us is loaded with them.

The terms "negative air ions" and "positive air ions" are, unfortunately, misleading, because negative charges are good for you and positive ones are not. In this case, "negative" and "positive" refer to the charge of the ion. So *negative ions = good; Positive ions = bad.*

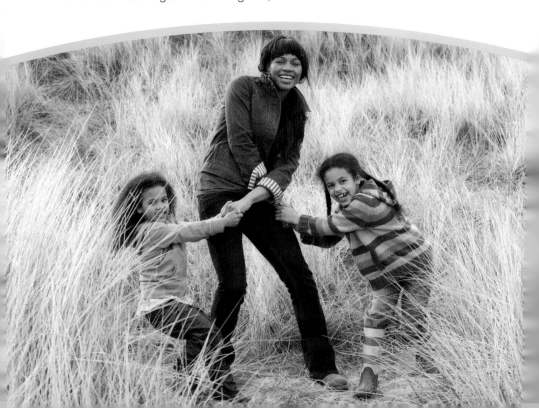

We'll pretend that the negative ions look like tiny *green* particles floating around and the positive ions look like tiny *red* ones. When looking through our Ion Detector Glasses, the particles suddenly become very visible. One of the first things we notice is that when we go outside, there are many more green dots than red ones in the air. Nature has far more negative charges than positive ones, which is a very good thing.

However, as soon as we step inside a typical home or building, the picture changes dramatically. Now we see a lot more red dots than green dots. Pollution and breathing the same air over and over depletes the negative ions. In our zeal to build energy efficient buildings, we have also sealed ourselves off from vital, fresh, outside air.

To get more negative ions in our system, we clearly need to spend more time outdoors and open windows to let the fresh air in. Another option is to possibly purchase an electronic device that may help purify the indoor air by generating negative ions.[112] Negative ions attract particles of pollution, such as dust, pollen, smoke and dander, giving them a negative charge. Those pollution particles then seek an electrical ground, which causes them to fall harmlessly to the floor. [113]

Certain indoor plants also help freshen the air by giving off negative ions.[114] NASA researchers have even demonstrated the effectiveness of using plants to deal with pollutants known to exist in spacecraft. Those same pollutants are present in homes and office buildings as well.[115]

Some of the benefits of negative ions:[116]

1. **Enhance mood.**
2. **Lower stress.**
3. **Stimulate appetite.**
4. **Boost energy.**
5. **Induce refreshing sleep.**
6. **Calm and invigorate the mind.**
7. **Protect against some germs in the air.**
8. **Improve alertness.**

Fresh air is one of God's precious gifts to us from our environment. It is vital to our health and well-being and has numerous benefits.

PRECIOUS GIFT #3 - SUNLIGHT

Sunlight is a third precious gift from God in our environment. Concerns that physicians have raised regarding the dangers of developing skin cancer from overexposure to the sun are certainly warranted. But that frightening prospect should not cause us to avoid proper and helpful exposure. Sunshine is one of God's healing agencies. With appropriate precautions, we all need adequate sunlight in order to maintain optimal health.

Ultraviolet radiation from the sun contains both UVA and UVB rays. Both can result in skin cancer. On the plus side of the equation, UVB is responsible for the production of vitamin D. Surveys indicate that many people today have vitamin D deficiency, which can put them at greater risk for problems such as osteoporosis, heart disease, and certain cancers other than skin cancer.[117] The amount of vitamin D that can be generated by sunlight depends on several factors such as where you live, age, diet, weight, skin color, and time of year.[118] Certain foods and vitamin D supplements are also potential sources.

Healthy exposure to sunlight can:[119]

1. **Lower blood pressure.**
2. **Eliminate toxins from the body.**
3. **Stave off Seasonal Affective Disorder (SAD).**
4. **Promote formation of serotonin and endorphins, which help regulate moods.**
5. **Stimulate the appetite.**
6. **Boost the immune system.**
7. **Enhance blood circulation.**
8. **Strengthen bones.**

Sunshine is one of God's healing agencies. With appropriate precautions, we all need adequate sunlight in order to maintain optimal health.

In Scripture, the three precious gifts – water, air, and light – are utilized by Jesus as images to describe himself and the blessings he longs to provide.

He is the only One who can quench our deep thirst for meaning and hope: "Jesus answered and said to her, 'Whoever drinks of this *water* will thirst again, but whoever drinks of the *water* that I shall give him will never thirst. But the *water* that I shall give him will become in him a fountain of *water* springing up into everlasting life'" (John 4:13-14, NKJV).

By receiving the Holy Spirit, we are taking in the life-giving breath of Christ himself. "So Jesus said to them again, 'Peace to you! As the Father has sent Me, I also send you.' And when He had said this, He *breathed* on them, and said to them, 'Receive the Holy Spirit'" (John 20:21-23, NKJV, emphasis added).

Jesus' life and teachings light the way to ultimate understanding and truth: "I have come into the world as a *light*, so that no one who believes in me should stay in darkness" (John 12:46 NIV, emphasis added).

God's three precious gifts from both the physical world and the spiritual realm are ours for the taking in order to fulfill his desire that we live life to the fullest.

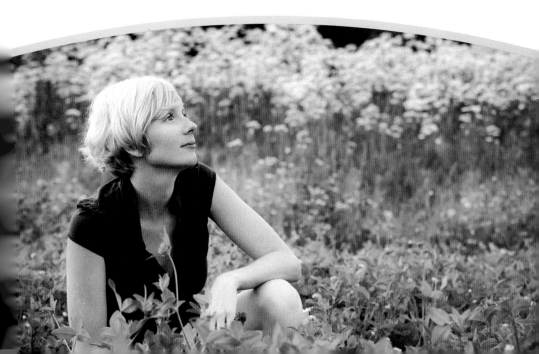

DISCUSSION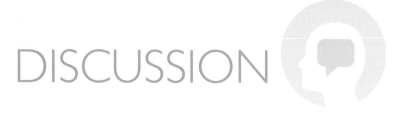

What is the coldest water you have ever been in? Describe your experience. Would you do it again?

....
....

Which type of water setting would you find most healing mentally and emotionally? Why?

OCEAN
....
RIVER
....
WATERFALL
....
TIDAL POOL
....
GEYSER
....

How would you try to convince a family member or friend that they needed to get more fresh air?

....
....

How could you bring more negative ions into your home or workplace?

....
....

Have you or someone you know ever experienced Seasonal Affective Disorder (SAD)? What impact did SAD have and what helped?

....
....

Why do you think Jesus used the act of drinking water to illustrate his ministry?

....
....

Describe an emotional or spiritual thirst in your life that Jesus is currently filling.

....
....

....

SHARING

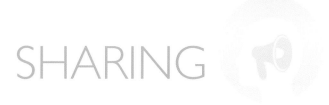

OPPORTUNITY #8:

- Pray for God to open the way for you to share something from these lessons to help someone else this week.

- Keep your radar up each day for opportunities.

ABUNDANT LIVING THOUGHT

To get more negative ions in our system, we clearly need to spend more time outdoors and open windows to let the fresh air in.

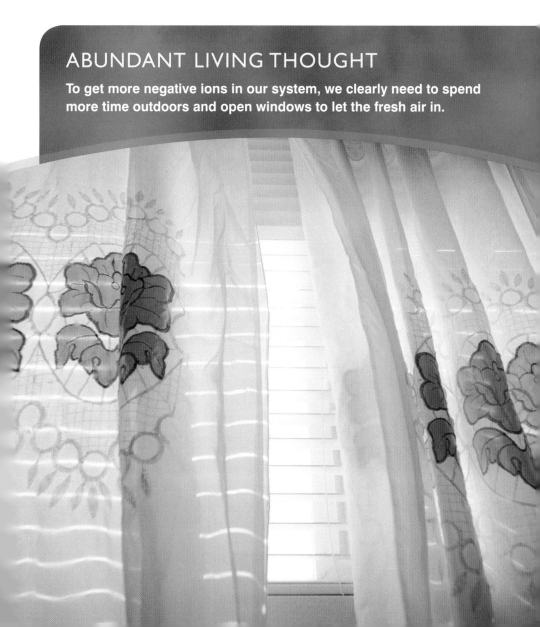

NOTES:

ABOUT THE AUTHOR

Kim Johnson is a popular writer, speaker, and fervent advocate for holistic living. As the author of three books, eleven lesson series, and many articles, his writings focus on healthy living and spiritual connectedness. His materials have been used in hundreds of churches throughout North America and internationally as well.

Johnson is an ordained minister with more than 35 years of experience as a parish pastor and church administrator. Over the years, his work with parishioners emphasized principles of whole-person health as a path to optimum mental, physical, social, and spiritual well-being. His later work with pastors and church leaders emphasized skill development such as vision casting, goal setting, support systems, relationship management, and accountability. Johnson has put his experience of working with pastors and parishioners to use in the CREATION Health Life Guide Series by creating a resource ideally suited for use in churches, small groups or individual study.

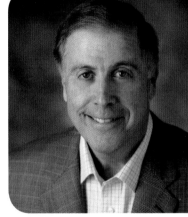

Johnson holds a Master of Divinity degree and received his Bachelor of Arts in theology. He currently serves as Director of Resource Development for churches in the state of Florida. His personal interests include reading, classical music, art and book festivals, kayaking, traveling, volunteering, and small group study. He and his wife Ann make their home in Orlando.

Author Acknowledgements: It has been a great privilege for me to be associated with the team of dedicated individuals who helped in various ways to make these CREATION Health Life Guides available. I would like to single out my wife Ann and daughter Stefanie, whose feedback and suggestions were always characterized by unfailing support and clear-eyed honesty. I have also received invaluable guidance and encouragement from Mike Cauley, Tim Nichols, Nick Howard, and Jim Epperson. Finally, I want to thank the group of local pastors who met with me personally and provided a wonderful forum for evaluating the lesson drafts.

NOTES

1. Edie West, *The Big Book of Icebreakers* (New York, NY: McGraw-Hill, 1999), 89.

2. Meryl Runion, *Perfect Phrases for Icebreakers* (New York, NY: McGraw-Hill, 2012), 2.

3. E. Merrill Root, http://thinkexist.com/quotations/wonder/3.html.

4. Brainy Quote, Jeanette Winterson, http://www.brainyquote.com/quotes/keywords/wonder_7.html.

5. "Inuit," http://en.wikipedia.org/wiki/Inuit; "Inuits of Greenland: An Adaptive Society," http://www.123helpme.com/view.asp?id=25880.

6. "Happiness Quotient - Astoundingly unhappy millionaires," October 19, 2007, http://blog.swash.org/2007/10/happiness-quotient-astoundingly-unhappy.html.

7. Michael Waldholz, "Garden Therapy," September 11, 2003, http://www.deseretnews.com/article/510053123/Garden-therapy-Just-looking-at-natural-vistas-may-help-improve-your-mental-physical-health.html ; Article – Nature and Nature Art, http://aliveltd.org/rspace/nature.html.

8. "Green Exercise," http://www.greenexercise.org/Green_Exercise.html.

9. Richard Louv, *The Nature Principle* (Chapel Hill, NC: Algonquin Books of Chapel Hill, 2011), 58-59.

10. Richard Louv, *The Nature Principle*, 111.

11. Richard Louv, *The Nature Principle*, 47.

12. Richard Louv, *The Nature Principle*, 33.

13. Richard Louv, *The Nature Principle,* 30.

14. Richard Louv, *The Nature Principle*, 30.

15. Richard Louv, *Last Child in the Woods* (Chapel Hill, NC: Algonquin Books of Chapel Hill, 2008), 51.

16. Richard Louv, *Last Child in the Woods*, 48.

17. Judy Molland, *Get Out!* (Minneapolis, MN: Free Spirit Publishing, 2009), 1-2.

18. Richard Louv, *The Nature Principle*, 254.

19. Children & Nature Network, http://www.childrenandnature.org/naturestory/; Richard Louv, *Last Child in the Woods,* 172.

20. Nature Quotations, Iris Murdoch, http://www.inspirational-quotations.com/nature-quotes.html.

21. Jerry D. Jones, 201 Great Questions (Colorado Spring, CO: NavPress, 1988), 18.

22. Garry Poole, *The Complete Book of Questions* (Grand Rapids, MI: Zondervan, 2003), 18.

23. Eva Shaw, PhD, *Shovel It* (Carlsbad, CA: Writeriffic Publishing Group, 2001), 1, 2, 9, 12.

24. Eva Shaw, PhD, *Shovel It*, 98-105.

25. Judy Molland, *Get Out!* (Minneapolis, MN: Free Spirit Publishing, 2009), 15.

26. Judy Molland, *Get Out!,* 16.

27. Judy Molland, *Get Out!,* 18.

28. Joseph Cornell, *Sharing Nature With Children* (Nevada City, CA: Dawn Publications, 1998), 22.

29. Joseph Cornell, *Sharing Nature With Children*, 27.

30. Joseph Cornell, *Sharing Nature With Children*, 48.

31. Joseph Cornell, *Sharing Nature With Children*, 50-51.

32. Joseph Cornell, *Sharing Nature With Children*, 58-59.

33. Joseph Cornell, *Sharing Nature With Children*, 75.

34. Richard Louv, *Last Child In the Woods*, 360.

35. Richard Louv, *Last Child In the Woods*, 362.

36. Jerry D. Jones, *201 Great Questions*, 16.

37. Deborah Branscum, "The Hoarding Syndrome - When Clutter Goes Out Of Control," *Reader's Digest*, March 2007, http://www.rd.com/health/the-hoarding-syndrome-when-clutter-goes-out-of-control/2/.

38. Nancy Twigg, *From Clutter to Clarity* (Cincinnati, OH: Standard Publishing, 2007), 109.

39. Nancy Twigg, *From Clutter to Clarity*, 112.

40. Sue Rasmussen, "Clear Your Clutter to Transform Your Life," http://www.unclutter-organize-transform.com/index.html.

41. Dr. Robin Zasio, *The Hoarder In You* (New York, NY: Rodale, 2011) 31-43; Amy Sung, "6 Types of Clutter & Why to Let Go,"February 11, 2011, http://clubspa.spafinder.com/wellness-week/types-clutter/ ; "Clutter 101: The Different Types Of Clutter," Apr 23, 2007, http://www.organizeit.co.uk/2007/04/23/clutter-101-the-different-types-of-clutter/ ; "Clutter 101: Why Do We Keep Clutter?" Mar 01, 2007, http://www.organizeit.co.uk/2007/03/01/clutter-101-why-do-we-keep-clutter/ ; Angie Kay, "My Minimalist Journey," July 17, 2011, http://minimalistwith3kids.blogspot.com/2011/07/types-of -clutter.http://minimalistwith3kids.blogspot.com/2011/07/types-of-clutter.html.

42. Dr. Robin Zasio, *The Hoarder In You*, 39.

43. "Clutter 101: Why Do We Keep Clutter?" Mar 01, 2007, http://www.organizeit.co.uk/2007/03/01/clutter-101-why-do-we-keep-clutter/.

44. Dr. Robin Zasio, *The Hoarder In You*, 37.

45. Dr. Robin Zasio, *The Hoarder In You*, 37, 42.

46. Amy Sung, "6 Types of Clutter & Why to Let It Go," February 11, 2011, http://clubspa.spafinder.com/wellness-week/types-clutter/.

47. Greg Hanson, "Clear Away the Clutter," December 2, 2007, http://www.sunriseonline.ca/sermons/clear_away_the_clutter.html; Karen Perkins, "Different Types of Clutter & How It Affects You," http://ezinearticles.com/?Different-Types-of-Clutter-and-How-it-Affects-You&id=2066466; Sue Rasmussen, "Why Stop Clutter?" http://www.unclutter-organize-transform.com/stop-clutter.html.

48. Barbara Ann Kipfer, *4,000 Questions for Getting to Know Anyone and Everyone* (New York, NY: Random House Reference, 2004), 80.

49. Garry Poole, *The Complete Book of Questions*, 121.

50. Jill Blake, *Healthy Home* (David & Charles Books, 1998), 77.

51. Geoffrey Montgomery, *"Breaking the Code of Color: How Do We See Colors?"* http://www.hhmi.org/senses/b110.html.

52. Frank H. Mahnke, *Color, Environment, and Human Response* (New York, NY: John Wiley & Sons, Inc, 1996), 6.

53. Jill Blake, *Healthy Home*, 84.

54. Frank H. Mahnke, *Color, Environment, and Human Response*, 94.

55. Ask Yahoo, December 27, 2004, http://ask.yahoo.com/20041227.html.

56. Jill Blake, *Healthy Home*, 84.

57. Marion Boddy-Evans, "What You Need to Know About Color Theory for Painting," http://painting.about.com/od/colourtheory/ss/color_theory.htm.

58. "Color Affects Mood," http://www.bhg.com/decorating/color/color-affects-mood/.

60. Leatrice Eiseman, *Pantone Guide to Communicating With Color* (Cincinnati, OH: HOW Books, 2000), 19.

60. Frank H. Mahnke, *Color, Environment, and Human Response*, 61; Leatrice Eiseman, *Pantone Guide to Communicating With Color,* 20.

61. Jill Blake, *Healthy Home*, 95.

62. "Room Color and How it Affects your Mood," http://freshome.com/2007/04/17/room-color-and-how-it-affects-your-mood/.

63. Jill Blake, *Healthy Home*, 92.

64. Frank H. Mahnke, *Color, Environment, and Human Response*, 63.

65. Frank H. Mahnke, *Color, Environment, and Human Response*, 73.

66. Leatrice Eiseman, Pantone Guide to Communicating With Color, 27-28.

67. "Room Color and How it Affects your Mood," http://freshome.com/2007/04/17/room-color-and-how-it-affects-your-mood/.

68. Jill Blake, *Healthy Home*, 78.

69. Meryl Runion, *Perfect Phrases for Icebreakers*, 51.

70. Barbara Ann Kipfer, *4,000 Questions for Getting to Know Anyone and Everyone*, 161.

71. John Albers, "How Does An Ear Work?" http://www.ehow.com/how-does_4563971_the-ear-work.html.

72. http://science.howstuffworks.com/environmental/life/human-biology/hearing.htm.

73. John Albers, "How Does An Ear Work?" http://www.ehow.com/how-does_4563971_the-ear-work.html.

74. http://science.howstuffworks.com/environmental/life/human-biology/hearing.htm.

75. Tom Harris, "How Hearing Works," http://science.howstuffworks.com/environmental/life/human-biology/hearing.htm.

76. Tom Harris, "How Hearing Works," http://science.howstuffworks.com/environmental/life/human-biology/hearing.htm.

77. Tom Harris, "How Hearing Works," http://science.howstuffworks.com/environmental/life/human-biology/hearing.htm.

78. Jeff Goldberg, "Signals From a Hair Cell," http://www.hhmi.org/senses/c110.html.

79. Jeff Goldberg, "Signals From a Hair Cell," http://www.hhmi.org/senses/c110.html.

80. Cindi Pearce, "Damaged Hair Cells of the Ear," http://www.ehow.com/list_7351878_damaged-hair-cells-ear.html.

81. "Decibel (Loudness) Comparison Chart," http://www.gcaudio.com/resources/howtos/loudness.html; Joshua Leeds, *The Power of Sound* (Rochester, VT: Healing Arts Press, 2010), 24.

82. Joshua Leeds, *The Power of Sound*, 84.

83. Jeff Goldberg, "Signals From a Hair Cell," http://www.hhmi.org/senses/c110.html.

84. Joshua Leeds, *The Power of Sound*, 90.

85. Manasi Chaudhari, "10 Benefits of Listening to Music," May 3, 2010, http://www.lifemojo.com/lifestyle/10-benefits-of-listening-to-music-19402577.

86. Don Campbell and Alex Doman, *Healing at Speed of Sound*, (London, England: Hudson Street Press, 2011) 103; Manasi Chaudhari, "10 Benefits of Listening to Music," May 3, 2010, http://www.lifemojo.com/lifestyle/10-benefits-of-listening-to-music-19402577 ; "Health Benefits of Listening to Music," November 15, 2010, http://www.medicaldaily.com/news/20101115/3740/health-benefits-of-listening-to-music.htm.

87. Don Campbell and Alex Doman, *Healing at the Speed of Sound,* 4.

88. Adam Ramsay, "Health benefits of music," http://www.netdoctor.co.uk/healthy-living/wellbeing/health-benefits-of-music.htm?fb_ref=fcbk.

89. Don Campbell and Alex Doman, *Healing at Speed of Sound*, 46, 68.

90. Joshua Leeds, *The Power of Sound*, 120.

91. Garry Poole, *The Complete Book of Questions*, 113.

92. Discovery Communications Inc., "Your Sense of Smell," 2000, http://yucky.discovery.com/flash/body/pg000150.html.

93. Gloria Rodriguez-Gil, MEd, "The Sense of Smell: A Powerful Sense," Spring 2004, http://www.tsbvi.edu/seehear/summer05/smell.htm.

94. Discovery Communications Inc., "Your Sense of Smell," 2000, http://yucky.discovery.com/flash/body/pg000150.html.

95. Sarah Dowdey, "How Smell Works," http://science.howstuffworks.com/environmental/life/human-biology/smell.htm.

96. "Scientists Win Nobel By A Nose," October 05, 2004, http://articles.orlandosentinel.com/keyword/sense-of-smell.

97. ScienceDaily, "Scientists Discover An Organizing Principle for Our Sense of Smell Based On Pleasantness," September 26, 2011, http://www.sciencedaily.com/releases/2011/09/110926104624.htm.

98. Sonu S., "How Does the Sense of Smell Work In Humans?" July 8, 2011, http://www.buzzle.com/articles/how-does-the-sense-of-smell-work-in-humans.html.

99. Sarah Dowdey, "How Smell Works," http://science.howstuffworks.com/environmental/life/human-biology/smell.htm.

100. Linda Andrews, "Scents make healthy sense," February 12, 2008, *Psychology Today* Magazine, http://articles.orlandosentinel.com/keyword/sense-of-smell.

101. Linda Andrews, "Scents make healthy sense," February 12, 2008, *Psychology Today* Magazine, http://articles.orlandosentinel.com/keyword/sense-of-smell.

102. Jill Blake, *Healthy Home*, 128.

103. Jill Blake, *Healthy Home*, 129.

104. Nicole Engel, "About Reed Diffusers," http://www.ehow.com/about_5101688_reed-diffusers.html.

105. Claire Jeffreys, "How to Use Herbs to Make Your House Smell Yummy," http://www.ehow.com/how_8361756_use-make-house-smell-yummy.html.

106. Yumi Sakugawa, "7 Ways to Make Your Living Space Smell Nice," May 3, 2011, http://www.care2.com/greenliving/diy-air-fresheners-7-ways-to-make-your-living-space-smell-nice.html.

107. "What's Really in That Luscious Chocolate Aroma?" *ScienceDaily*, Aug. 29, 2011, http://www.sciencedaily.com/releases/2011/08/110829142510.htm.

108. "Benefits of Hydrotherapy," http://www.watertechtn.com/hydrotherapy.htm; "Water: A Powerful Potential For Healing," http://www.healthy100.org/water-powerful-potential-healing; "Hot baths are good for your health,"

http://just-healthy.net/hot-baths ; "Health Benefits of a Bath," http://www.sunflowernaturals.com/article_bath_benefits.shtml.

109. "Contrast Shower," http://www.natural-health-restored.com/contrast-shower.html.

110. Jackie Frederick, "An Epidemic Checked: A Chronicle of the 1918 Influenza Pandemic in Dayton, Ohio," 2003, http://www.daytonhistorybooks.com/page/page/2753646.htm.

111. Ronda Smith, "Start Breathing," October 29, 2010, http://www.newstart.com/blog/start-breathing/#more-839.

112. Jim English, "The Positive Health Benefits of Negative Ions," http://www.nutritionreview.org/library/negative.ions.php.

113. *"What Are Negative and Positive Ions? How do they work?"* http://www.microncorp.com/energaire/ions.html.

114. "A Dozen Plants that Clean Indoor Air," http://lifehacker.com/5557235/a-dozen-more-plants-for-better-indoor-air.

115. Laura Pottorrf, "Plants 'Clean' Air Inside Our Homes," http://www.colostate.edu/Depts/CoopExt/4DMG/Plants/clean.htm.

116. Celeste Lee, "Open Air," http://www.lifestylelaboratory.com/articles/open-air.html; "Get A Breath of Fresh Air!" http://www.natural-health-restored.com/fresh-air.html; "Effects of Negative Ions," http://www.peakpureair.com/effects-negative-ions; Denise Mann, "Negative Ions Create Positive Vibes," WebMd, 5-6-2002, http://www.webmd.com/balance/features/negative-ions-create-positive-vibes.

117. Deborah Kotz, "Time in the Sun: How Much Is Needed for Vitamin D?" June 23, 2008, http://health.usnews.com/health-news/family-health/heart/articles/2008/06/23/time-in-the-sun-how-much-is-needed-for-vitamin-d.

118. "How Much Sunshine or Vitamin D do I Need? What Vitamin D Dosage?" http://www.healthdiscoveries.net/vitamin-D.html.

119. Richard Hobday PhD, *The Healing Sun* (Scotland, UK: Findhord Press, 1999), 22; Payal Banka, "Health Benefits of Sunlight," July 24, 2010, http://www.lifemojo.com/lifestyle/health-benefits-of-sunlight-35071756 ; "Benefits of Sunlight," http://www.natural-health-restored.com/benefits-of-sunlight.html ; Suzanna Hulmes, "Benefits of Sunlight," http://www.ehow.com/list_7214325_benefits-sunlight.html ; "Sunlight," http://newstartclub.com/resources/detail/sunlight1.

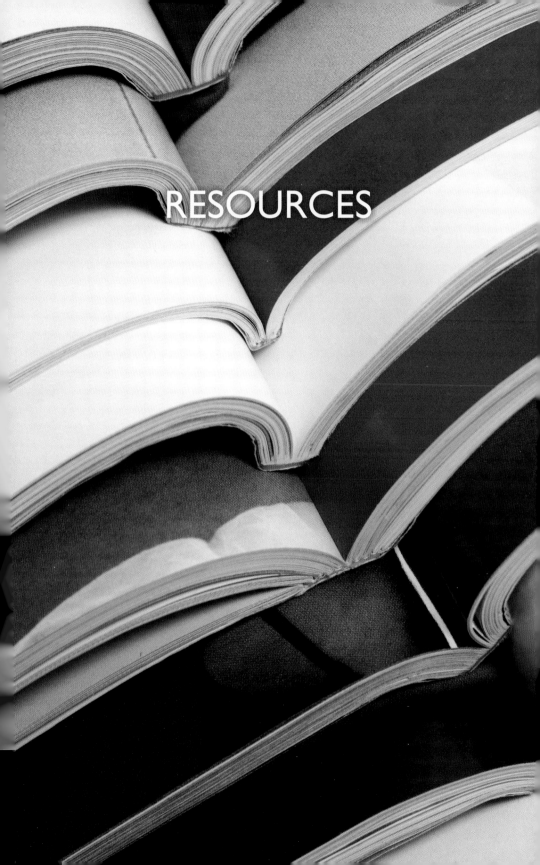
RESOURCES

LEAD YOUR COMMUNITY
TO HEALTHY
LIVING

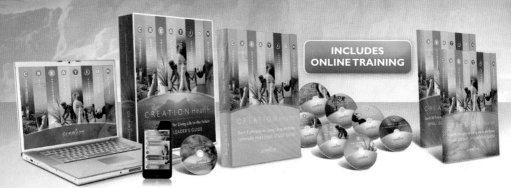

INCLUDES ONLINE TRAINING

Seminar Leader Kit

Everything a leader needs to conduct this seminar successfully, including key questions to facilitate group discussion and PowerPoint presentations for each of the eight principles.

Participant Guide

A study guide with essential information from each of the eight lessons along with outlines, self assessments, and questions for people to fill-in as they follow along.

Small Group Kit

It's easy to lead a small group using the CREATION Health videos, the Small Group Leaders Guide and the Small Group Discussion Guide.

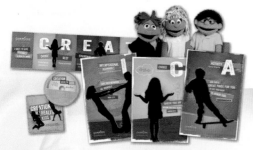

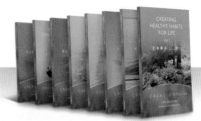

CREATION Kids

CREATION Health Kids can make a big difference in homes, schools and congregations. Lead kids in your community to healthier, happier living.

Life Guide Series

These guides include questions designed to help individuals or small groups study the depths of every principle and learn strategies for integrating them into everyday life.

GUIDES AND ASSESSMENTS

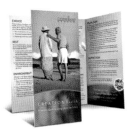

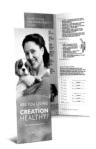

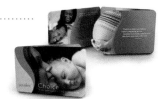

Pregnancy Guides
Expert advice on how to be CREATION Healthy while expecting.

Senior Guide
Share the CREATION Health principles with seniors and help them be healthier and happier as they live life to the fullest.

Self-Assessment
This instrument raises awareness about how CREATION Healthy a person is in each of the eight major areas of wellness.

Pocket Guide
A tool for keeping people committed to living all of the CREATION Health principles daily.

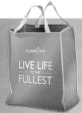

Tote Bag
A convenient way for bringing CREATION Health materials to and from class.

Water Bottle
Practice good Nutrition and keep yourself hydrated with the CREATION Health water bottle.

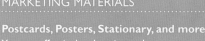

MARKETING MATERIALS

Postcards, Posters, Stationary, and more
You can effectively advertise and generate community excitement about your CREATION Health seminar with a wide range of available marketing materials such as enticing postcards, flyers, posters, and more.

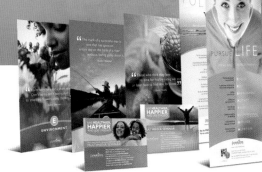

Bible Stories
God is interested in our physical, mental and spiritual well being. Throughout the Bible you can discover the eight principles for full life.

CREATION HEALTH BOOKS

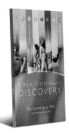

CREATION Health Discovery
Written by Des Cummings, Jr., PhD and Monica Reed, MD, this wonderful companion resource introduces people to the CREATION Health philosophy and lifestyle.

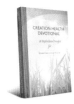

CREATION Health Devotional
In this devotional you will discover stories about experiencing God's grace in the tough times, God's delight in triumphant times, and God's presence in peaceful times.

English: Hardcover
Spanish: Softcover

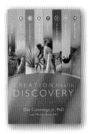

CREATION Health Discovery (Softcover)

CREATION Health Discovery takes the 8 essential principles of CREATION Health and melds them together to form the blueprint for the health we yearn for and the life we are intended to live.

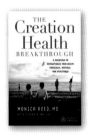

CREATION Health Breakthrough (Hardcover)

Blending science and lifestyle recommendations, Monica Reed, MD, prescribes eight essentials that will help reverse harmful health habits and prevent disease. Discover how intentional choices, rest, environment, activity, trust, relationships, outlook, and nutrition can put a person on the road to wellness. Features a three-day total body rejuvenation therapy and four-phase life transformation plan.

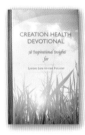

CREATION Health Devotional (English: Hardcover / Spanish: Softcover)

Stories change lives. Stories can inspire health and healing. In this devotional you will discover stories about experiencing God's grace in the tough times, God's delight in triumphant times, and God's presence in peaceful times. Based on the eight timeless principles of wellness: Choice, Rest, Environment, Activity, Trust, Interpersonal relationships, Outlook, Nutrition.

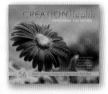

CREATION Health Devotional for Women (English)

Written for women by women, the *CREATION Health Devotional for Women* is based on the principles of whole-person wellness represented in CREATION Health. Spirits will be lifted and lives rejuvenated by the message of each unique chapter. This book is ideal for women's prayer groups, to give as a gift, or just to buy for your own edification and encouragement.

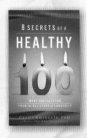

8 Secrets of a Healthy 100 (Softcover)

Can you imagine living to a Healthy 100 years of age? Dr. Des Cummings Jr., explores the principles practiced by the All-stars of Longevity to live longer and more abundantly. Take a journey through the 8 Secrets and you will be inspired to imagine living to a Healthy 100.

Forgive To Live (English: Hardcover / Spanish: Softcover)

In Forgive to Live Dr. Tibbits presents the scientifically proven steps for forgiveness – taken from the first clinical study of its kind conducted by Stanford University and Florida Hospital.

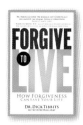

Forgive To Live Workbook (Softcover)

This interactive guide will show you how to forgive – insight by insight, step by step – in a workable plan that can effectively reduce your anger, improve your health, and put you in charge of your life again, no matter how deep your hurts.

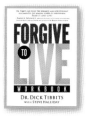

Forgive To Live Devotional (Hardcover)

In his powerful new devotional Dr. Dick Tibbits reveals the secret to forgiveness. This compassionate devotional is a stirring look at the true meaning of forgiveness. Each of the 56 spiritual insights includes motivational Scripture, an inspirational prayer, and two thought-provoking questions. The insights are designed to encourage your journey as you begin to *Forgive to Live*.

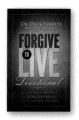

Forgive To Live God's Way (Softcover)

Forgiveness is so important that our very lives depend on it. Churches teach us that we should forgive, but how do you actually learn to forgive? In this spiritual workbook noted author, psychologist, and ordained minister Dr. Dick Tibbits takes you step-by-step through an eight-week forgiveness format that is easy to understand and follow.

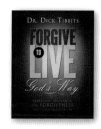

Forgive To Live Leader's Guide

Perfect for your community, church, small group or other settings.

The Forgive to Live Leader's Guide Includes:

- 8 Weeks of pre-designed PowerPoint™ presentations.
- Professionally designed customizable marketing materials and group handouts on CD-Rom.
- Training directly from author of Forgive to Live Dr. Dick Tibbits across 6 audio CDs.
- Media coverage DVD.
- CD-Rom containing all files in digital format for easy home or professional printing.
- A copy of the first study of its kind conducted by Stanford University and Florida Hospital showing a link between decreased blood pressure and forgiveness.

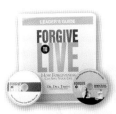

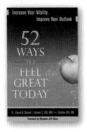

52 Ways to Feel Great Today (Softcover)

Wouldn't you love to feel great today? Changing your outlook and injecting energy into your day often begins with small steps. In *52 Ways to Feel Great Today*, you'll discover an abundance of simple, inexpensive, fun things you can do to make a big difference in how you feel today and every day. Tight on time? No problem. Each chapter is written as a short, easy-to-implement idea. Every idea is supported by at least one true story showing how helpful implementing the idea has proven to someone a lot like you. The stories are also included to encourage you to be as inventive, imaginative, playful, creative, or adventuresome as you can.

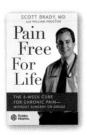

Pain Free For Life (Hardcover)

In *Pain Free For Life*, Scott C. Brady, MD, – founder of Florida Hospital's Brady Institute for Health – shares for the first time with the general public his dramatically successful solution for chronic back pain, Fibromyalgia, chronic headaches, Irritable bowel syndrome and other "impossible to cure" pains. Dr. Brady leads pain-racked readers to a pain-free life using powerful mind-body-spirit strategies used at the Brady Institute – where more than 80 percent of his chronic-pain patients have achieved 80-100 percent pain relief within weeks.

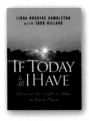

If Today Is All I Have (Softcover)

At its heart, Linda's captivating account chronicles the struggle to reconcile her three dreams of experiencing life as a "normal woman" with the tough realities of her medical condition. Her journey is punctuated with insights that are at times humorous, painful, provocative, and life-affirming.

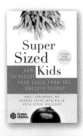

SuperSized Kids (Hardcover)

In *SuperSized Kids*, Walt Larimore, MD, and Sherri Flynt, MPH, RD, LD, show how the mushrooming childhood obesity epidemic is destroying children's lives, draining family resources, and pushing America dangerously close to a total healthcare collapse – while also explaining, step by step, how parents can work to avert the coming crisis by taking control of the weight challenges facing every member of their family.

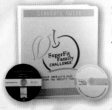

SuperFit Family Challenge – Leader's Guide

Perfect for your community, church, small group or other settings.

The SuperFit Family Challenge Leader's Guide Includes:

- 8 Weeks of pre-designed PowerPoint™ presentations.
- Professionally designed marketing materials and group handouts from direct mailers to reading guides.
- Training directly from Author Sherri Flynt, MPH, RD, LD, across 6 audio CDs.
- Media coverage and FAQ on DVD.

LIVE YOUR LIFE
TO THE FULLEST

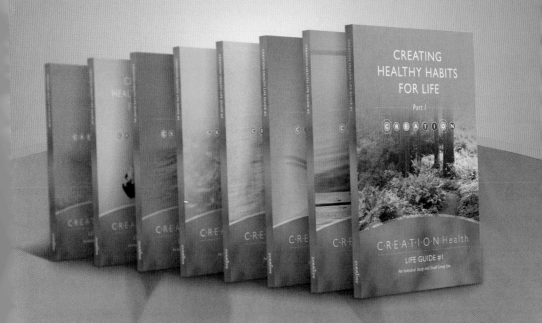

C·R·E·A·T·I·O·N Health

LIFE GUIDE SERIES

8 Guides. 8 Principles. One Powerful Message.
Packed with fresh insights on abundant living.
For Individual Study and Small Group Use.

Perfect for churches, schools, universities, and faith-based businesses.

IMAGINE...
A body that is healthy and strong,
A spirit that is vibrant and refreshed,
A life that glorifies God,
Imagine living to a **Healthy 100**.

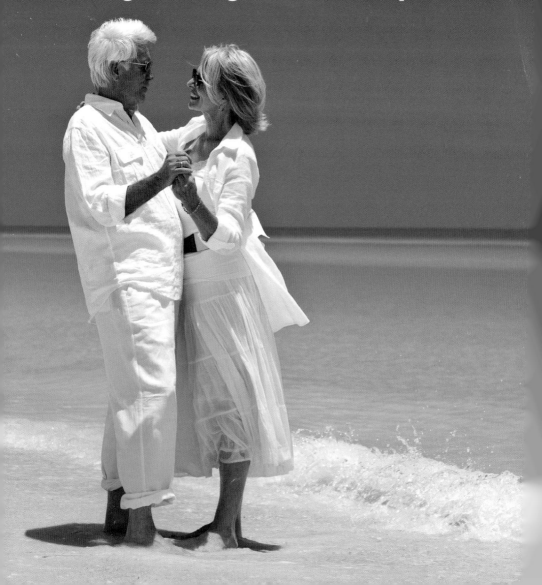